Anticipating and Assessing Health Care Technology Volume 3

Scenario Commission on Future
Health Care Technology

chairman H. David Banta

senior researcher Annetine Gelijns

Anticipating and Assessing Health Care Technology Volume 3

Developments in the Regeneration, Repair and Reorganization of Nervous Tissue

A report, commissioned by the
Steering Committee on Future Health Scenarios

1988
Kluwer Academic Publishers
Dordrecht – Boston – London

Distributors

for the United States and Canada: Kluwer Academic Publishers.
101 Philip Drive, Norwell, MA 02061, U.S.A.
For all other countries: Kluwer Academic Publishers Group,
P.O. Box 322, 3300 AH Dordrecht, The Netherlands

Steering Committee
on Future Health Scenarios
P.O. Box 5406
2280 HK Rijswijk
The Netherlands
Telephone: 070-407209

ISBN 0-89838-419-2

PRINTED IN THE NETHERLANDS.

Foreword

This report, **Developments in the Regeneration, Repair and Reorganization of Nervous Tissue**, is the third report from the STG Commission on Future Health Care Technology and one of a series of case studies from that project. It focuses on future applications of neurosciences, especially regarding Alzheimer's disease, Parkinson's disease, and accidents involving nervous system trauma. The STG (Stuurgroep Toekomstscenario's Gezondheidzorg) was established in 1983 as an independent advisory group to the State Secretary for Welfare, Public Health, and Cultural Affairs (WVC) to assist in long-range health planning efforts. Thus far, STG commissions have examined cardiovascular disease, cancer, aging, and life styles as issues of importance to the health of the Dutch population in the future.

Obviously, health care technology is of great concern to the government. On the one hand, technology is one of the major tools to promote a healthy population. On the other hand, the costs of health care have been rising at an alarming rate in recent years. It was these two facts, along with the social consequences of certain technologies such as genetic screening, that led the STG to establish the Commission on Future Health Care Technology in 1985. The European Office of the World Health Organization (EURO) cosponsored the project. The Health Council (Gezondheidsraad) agreed to cooperate with the project by furnishing space and intellectual and logistical support.

The goal of the Commission's work is to develop sufficient information on future technological developments in health and health care to assist planning for their consequences.

The first report, **Anticipating and Assessing Health Care Technology**, gave the overall context for activities concerning future health care technology. The government and Dutch society as a whole must move rapidly to deal with the consequences of technological change in health care. The first report provided conclusions for achieving this purpose, focusing on the need to develop a national program or system of health care technology assessment.

The second report, **Future Technological Changes**, presented detailed information on anticipated future health care technologies. In the context of STG's studies, this might be considered an 'early warning system' for health care technology.

The fourth report, being published simultaenously, is **Health Care Applications of Lasers: The Future Treatment of Coronary Artery Disease**. It presents a general introduction to lasers in health care, although more detailed information is presented in Volume II. The main purpose of this case study is to examine the possible impacts of one application of lasers: the treatment of coronary artery disease.

The fifth report, **Developments in Genetic Testing**, examines another application of the new biotechnology, the rapidly developing field of genetics. The genetic revolution has now truly begun and it will transform the ways that society deals with its genetic inheritance. The implications of this new technology are far-reaching. The report explores some of these implications and suggests the importance of careful monitoring of this field.

The sixth report, **Applications of the New Biotechnology: The Case of Vaccines**, discusses developments in the new biotechnology. The ability to directly manipulate the genetic structure of organisms has lead to dramatic changes in biological research, and is now beginning to transform practical technology as well. The report presents some of the new developments in diagnostic and therapeutic technologies. The main purpose of the report, however, is to point out the potential applications in vaccine development and possible future impacts of this field on the health of the Netherlands population.

The seventh report, **Computer Assisted Medical Imaging: The Case of Picture Archiving and Communications Systems (PACS)**, presents information on an important new technology. Since the early 1970s, departments of radiology have gradually turned to imaging with computers, and there are now predictions that all medical images, including conventional x-rays, will be computerized. Such a move would have great potential advantages, but the costs to the health care system and society would also be large. It is important for Dutch society to become aware of these developments and to determine the best course of future action.

The final report from the project on future health care technology, **Potentials for Home Care Technology**, gives an overview of present and future developments in an important and often-neglected field of health care. The report also describes and analyses the home care system of the Netherlands, and conlcudes that the home care system is not structured to be receptive to technology. Therefore, the report suggests ways that the home care system could be improved.

As Chairman of the STG, I am delighted to present this report, and I thank the Commission very sincerely for its rapid and excellent work. The government expects to see changes in policies toward health care technology, and I am certain that the report will be a substantial help in that process of change.

The report was prepared by the Commission's staff, which is listed in this report. The staff was led by Dr. David Banta, an American who agreed to spend two years with the STG chairing the Commission. The decision to invite Dr. Banta to the Netherlands was a recognition of the international nature of issues concerning health care technology. I would also like to point out the presence of a Swede, Dr. Henry Danielson, and a Belgian, Professor Jan Blanpain, on the Commission. Dr. Johannes Vang from WHO/EURO was an official observer on the Commission. We are particularly grateful to these outside guests.

The reports have been developed with the help of experts and reviewed by the Commission and by many other individuals and groups representing a wide range of disciplines and perspectives. We are grateful for their many contributions. As with all STG reports, however, the content of the report is the responsibility of the Commission and the STG and does not necessarily represent the position of any of those who assisted or of the Ministry of WVC.

J. van Londen
Chairman, STG

Preface

As noted in the Foreword, this report is one of several volumes resulting from this study of future health care technology.

The purpose of the study, as formulated by the STG, was to analyze future health care technology. Part of the task was to develop an 'early warning system' for health care technology. The primary goal of the project was to develop a list or description of a number of possible and probable future health care technologies, as well as information on their importance. Within the limits of time and money, this has been done. However, given the vast number of possible future health care technologies, complete information on the importance of each area could not be developed in any depth for all technology.

Therefore, four specific technologies were chosen and were prospectively assessed. These future technologies were examined in more depth, looking particularly at their future health and policy implications. Subsequently, the project was extended to September 1986, and two additional technologies will be assessed.

The total output of the project is as follows:

Volume 1. GENERAL CONSIDERATIONS AND POLICY RECOMMENDATIONS

Volume 2. FUTURE TECHNOLOGICAL CHANGES

Volume 3. DEVELOPMENTS IN THE REGENERATION, REPAIR AND REORGANIZATION OF NERVOUS TISSUE

Volume 4. HEALTH CARE APPLICATIONS OF LASERS: The future treatment of coronary artery disease

Volume 5. DEVELOPMENTS IN GENETIC TESTING

Volume 6. APPLICATIONS OF THE NEW BIOTECHNOLOGY: The case of vaccines

Volume 7. COMPUTER-ASSISTED MEDICAL IMAGING: The Case of Picture Archiving and Communications Systems (PACS)

Volume 8. POTENTIALS FOR HOME CARE TECHNOLOGY

The first report was addressed to an important purpose. The Commission reached the tentative conclusion early in its deliberations that a system for identifying future health care technology would be of limited benefit on its own. The Netherlands does not have an organized system for technology assessment in health care, and therefore information on the benefits, risks, financial costs, and social implications of technology is not available for new or established technology, generally speaking. The Commission saw the need for such a system. Studies aimed at the identification and assessment of future health care technologies must be developed within such a context, the Commission concluded. Therefore, Volume I was developed as an overall policy document, and contains summary material on future technologies. This report gives the detailed information on the same technologies and technological areas.

The second report presented overall information on future health care technology. The report was based on information obtained from surveys done in the United States and in Europe.

The case studies are intended to examine important areas of future (and emerging) health care technology. However, many other potential subjects and applications could be examined. This case study, then, is only an example of what may be possible in evaluating the impacts of future health care technology.

Technological developments in health care are occurring rapidly, and the information on future technologies in these report will rapidly become out-of-date. The Commission is aware of this fact, and hopes that it will be possible to continue an 'early warning system' that will periodically update such information and assess specific technologies.

This report is primarily addressed to policy makers and to those who are interested in national level policy making. At the same time, the Commission believes that the information in this report is an important basis for future activities in health care technology assessment in Netherlands and in other countries.

Dr. H. David Banta
Chairman
Commission on Future Health Care Technology

Drs. Annetine Gelijns
Case Study Director

Table of Contents

Introduction

The quest for knowledge about the biological basis of human nature, especially the inquiry into man's brain, is one of the most complex challenges in science. Understanding the functioning of the central nervous system (brain and spinal cord) sheds light on fundamental questions of human nature and will lead to better ways of approaching the health-related problems involving the nervous system.

Neurosciences is the scientific field which investigates the development, organization, and operation of the nervous system. It focuses on the mechanisms underlying normal and abnormal behavior. Although knowledge concerning the central nervous system has been accumulating over centuries, it appears to be evolving even more rapidly at present. For example, in the 1940s, 1950s, and 1960s new techniques in anatomy (electron microscopy) and physiology (electrical recording) revealed the structure and functioning of the basic building blocks of the nervous system: nerve cells and the synapses (connections) between them. During the past two decades, other technical innovations, such as those in cell biology or in medical imaging, have brought further significant advances.

The study of the highly complex anatomical and functional structure of the nervous system is necessary to gain further insight into the basic mechanisms involved in neurological, communicative, and behavioral disorders. However, to date, the basic mechanisms underlying these disorders are still largely unknown. Ultimately, an increasing understanding of the functioning of the brain may also reveal the basis of such mental processes as memory, feelings, and cognition.

Nervous system disorders which include, among others, dementia, psychoses, affective disorders, multiple sclerosis and addiction afflict a significant part of the population (Table 1). Most of them are chronic and dehumanizing diseases, which cause an immense amount of suffering of both the afflicted individuals and their families, as well as raising societal issues such as the need for and cost of care and support. Those afflicted generally have physical problems, such as decreased mobility, and they may also have intellectual and psychological problems. The wide range of deficits associated with these diseases can also cause social problems for those afflicted.

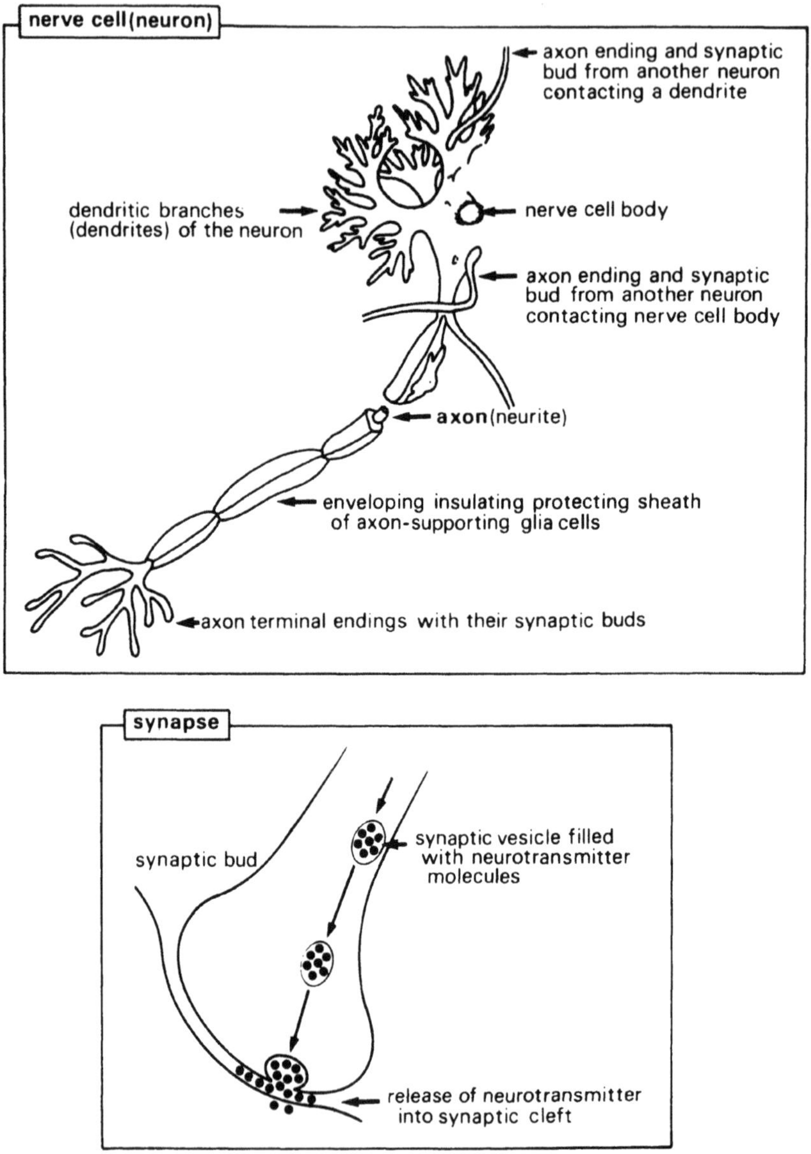

Figure 1 Nerve Cell and Synapse

Table 1 Estimated prevalence of a number of neurological, psychiatric and communicative disorders, The Netherlands, 1985

Disorders	Approximately
Dementia (over 65)	117.000
Parkinson's disease	28.000
Accidents, resulting in Central Nervous System Trauma	40.000
Demyelinating diseases (Multiple Sclerosis)	14.000
Convulsive disorders (e.g. epilepsy)	100.000
Alcoholism and Drug Dependance	650.000
Deafness	20.000
Seriously impaired hearing	400.000
Blindness	25.000
Seriously impaired vision	75.000
Aphasia	21.000
Brain tumors	15.000
Stroke*	150.000
Psychosis (e.g. schizophrenia)*	150.000
Mental retardation due to congenital defects or birth injuries*	150.000

* Obtained by adjusting US data for the difference in population
Source: (29)

From the public point of view, these disorders drain both public and private resources. Furthermore, many of the neurodegenerative and communicative disorders are correlated with age. Their prevalence thus can be projected to rise in the future due to the aging of the population.

If one takes into account the present and future prevalence of neurological, communicative, and behavioral disorders, future improvements in prevention, diagnosis, and treatment will benefit numerous people. As a considerable number of these people are institutionalized the inhabitants of nursing homes consist predominantly of patients with dementia and stroke the implications of improved prevention and treatment for the delivery and organization of health care are apparent.

New technological applications of neurosciences research will give rise to public policy issues in the future. A prospective assessment of possible new technologies may help policy makers to anticipate such issues and subsequently to improve decision making. The need for prospective assessment is highlighted if one considers the accelerating pace of advance in neurosciences.

As neurosciences is such a vast field, an in-depth assessment could only be done of part of it. The Working Group on Neurosciences suggested the case of the regeneration, repair, and reorganization of central and peripheral nervous tissue for in-depth analysis. The phenomena of regeneration, repair, and reorgnization of nervous tissue are generally a reflection of the dynamic properties or **plasticity** of nervous tissue. In this case the focus is on the **probabilities** resulting from plasticity research for improvements in prevention and treatment of certain diseases and disorders. These include Alzheimer's disease, Parkinson's disease, and accidents involving nervous system trauma. In addition to future health implications, effects on the delivery of care as well as broader social consequences may be expected. The presently developing techniques, for example, involve major ethical implications, such as the possibility of using fetal tissue in brain grafting. Consequences for the delivery of care can be found, for instance, in a potential delay of the onset of dementia for 5 years. Such a delay would decrease the number of demented persons in Dutch nursing homes by 26% up to the year 2000, in comparison with a no-change scenario (120). Such potential implications will be addressed in this case-study.

The **organization** of the report is as follows. In the first chapter of the report, some examples of promising directions of neurosciences research are provided to illustrate the rapid advances in this field as well as the questions raised by these advances. The second chapter reviews developments in plasticity research and its potential future technological applications. Chapters III and IV analyze future applications of such research for health and health care, as well as broader social implications. The report is concluded with brief policy conclusions and an indication of the resources needed for the implementation of these conclusions.

Chapter I – Some Promising Directions of Research and Technology Development in Neurosciences

"If the human brain would be so simple that we could understand it, we would be so simple that we couldn't".

The brain and nervous system are involved in sensation, motion, regulation of internal biological processes, reproduction, and adaptation to the external world. Many aspects of human functioning, such as perception, movement, emotion, thought, and memory, result from highly intricate patterns of activity within the brain (15). Dysfunctioning of the brain and nervous system can lead to a wide array of neurological, communicative, and behavioral disorders. These disorders include developmental defects, learning handicaps, sensory deficits, depressive conditions, schizophrenia, multiple sclerosis, and neurological deficits due to injuries. Some of them can be particularly dehumanizing, as they lead to a deterioration in essential human functions, such as the ability to communicate with others. The functioning and dysfunctioning of the central nervous system in general involve fundamental questions of human nature.

As mentioned above, neurosciences is the scientific field that investigates the development, organization,and operation of the nervous system. It focuses on the mechanisms underlying normal and abnormal behavior. The goal of neurosciences is to define and understand the continuum from molecule to cell, from cell to nervous system, and from nervous system to behavior (99). The brain consists of approximately one hundred billion highly specialized cells, called neurons. These neurons communicate with each other by conducting electrical information along their cell membranes and transferring this information from one cell to another by means of chemical messengers (chemical neurotransmitters), or via direct electrical signals.

One of the basic tenets in neurosciences is that human behavior and mental activity ultimately originate in electrical and chemical events in circuits of neurons. The interaction between endogenous and environmental factors also plays a major role in brain function. As in all health-related problems, the central issue is this interaction between endogenous (biological) factors on the one hand and environmental factors on the other. Or, in other words, an optimal relationship between the central nervous system, the organism as a whole, and its environment is vital to health and survival.

At present the area of neurosciences research is rapidly evolving. At the cellular level, new techniques in the field of molecular genetics and biochemistry, for instance, are producing new fundamental information on the elements that make up the nervous system. At the level of large populations of nerve cells, insight is beginning to emerge how behavior is organized and controlled. At this level, multidisciplinary research involving neuroscientists, ethologists, psychologists, and computer scientists, is emerging. Advances in these areas provide further steps in unraveling the complex brain-behavior relationship. This Chapter presents some examples of recent achievements, and prospects for future progress out of the vast area of neurosciences research.

Genetic Factors

Some disorders of the central nervous system, for instance those resulting in mental retardation[1], are known to be of genetic (inherited) origin (75).

For a few dozen genetic neurological disorders, the responsible (enzyme) protein defect has been elucidated. In some instances, as in phenylketonuria, it has been possible to develop a screening test and to design a dietary treatment whereby mental retardation can be prevented. In most cases, however, understanding of the molecular etiology has not yet resulted in therapeutic approaches mainly because of biological difficulties, including the blood brain barrier (see brief on this subject) (4; 7).

Recently, the gene responsible for Huntington's disease (or Huntington's Chorea) has been localized. Huntington's disease is a serious, inherited, and eventually lethal neurological disease (86).

---

[1]) Approximately 25 percent of the causes of mental retardation are of genetic origin (Gezondheidsraad, 1985).

It involves progressive loss of movement and of intellectual and psychological impairment. The disease usually manifests itself around the 40th year of life, often after the genetic defect has been passed on to children. The children thus must wait until their late middle age before being reasonably certain that they will not develop the disease themselves. There is no therapy for the disease. The identification of the abnormal gene has now made possible a predictive test for people at risk. This genetic probe has only been used for research and still has certain technical limitations, but clinical application of the predictive test is now being considered. This leads to a number of complex ethical and legal issues, such as whether people should be tested during pregnancy or at birth, and whether they should be told that they do or do not have the gene.

In addition to these real Mendelian (inherited) neurological disorders, genetic factors seem to play a major role in the etiology of a number of nervous system disorders, including the psychoses such as schizophrenia and the affective disorders (e.g. depressive illness). Important progress has been achieved in the study of such diseases at the (sub-)cellular level during the last decades. The application of molecular biology has, for example, resulted in a growing number of genetic markers[2]. These genetic markers can be used to identify and isolate genes, shown to play a central etiological role in certain nervous system disorders (96).

Research is also being carried out in the field of a number of other diseases. For example, there are attempts to find a gene for Alzheimer's disease as well as a genetic marker (76). In multiple sclerosis (MS), an association has been found between the disease and genes in an area of the 6th chromosome responsible for regulating the immune response, indicating that there may be a link between immunological abnormalities and onset of this disease.

In the future, information obtained through the use of recombinant DNA methods will be valuable for the diagnosis of inherited neurological or behavioral disorders and for genetic counselling of

---

[2]) A genetic marker is a measurable or observable signpost or signal of the presence or location of a gene, chromosome, or hereditary characteristic. Observation that one is of the male sex, for example, is a reliable indicator of the presence of the gene for H-Y antigen, a cell surface protein found in all those who are genetically male.

those at risk. Subsequently, the potential to isolate and characterize significant genes could result in a better understanding of the physical basis of disease and thus lead to new approaches in treatment (96).

As mentioned above, however, the use of genetic markers will also give rise to important ethical and legal issues. Ethical issues can be roughly divided into those: concerning the accuracy of the test and the possibility of inaccurate predictions;

- concerning the burden of this knowledge for the individual in case the identification of a gene is made;
- concerning potential social consequences and stigmatization, such as changes in job selection procedures or in solidarity patterns in national insurance (33).

These ethical issues will have to be dealt with and guidelines need to be established.

Communication in the Nervous System

Brain functioning and nerve cell communication depend on interacting chemical and electrical processes. Crucial functions of nerve cell communication are associated with, and are dependent on, the flow of electrical currents. Electrical currents are carried by ions across the cell membrane through so-called ion channels.

Recently, new electrophysiological and biochemical techniques have advanced the understanding of ion channel related processes. Even rather subtle changes in the general properties of one or several types of ion channels might produce far-reaching alterations in nervous functions. Disturbances of this class of cellular properties are likely to be involved in several kinds of neurological or psychiatric diseases for which the precise etiology is still unclear.

An example of such a disease is epilepsy. In the Netherlands, a general practitioner with a clinical practice of 2000 people will, on average, find 14 patients suffering from epilepsy (89). Recently, new insights in the genesis of epilepsy have been obtained at the basic physiological level. Epilepsy is a collection of clinical manifestations which have as a common denominator the occurrence of seizures. At the cellular level, a large number of nerve cells discharge during an epileptic seizure.

New insights have been mainly acquired in experimental models of epilepsy in intact animals (in vivo) (84), combined with new techniques that enable brain tissue to be kept functional outside the animal in an appropriate medium (in vitro). The ion conductivities of the membranes of neurons invoved in an epileptogenic focus (an abnormal focus that seems to initiate the seizure) are being studied. The conditions for the production of a chain reaction of excitation which spreads over a whole neuronal network have been analysed in detail. Changes in ion concentrations and other electrophysiological aspects of brain functioning are being intensively investigated. Mathematical models of neuronal networks are being used to clarify the role of different cellular and synaptic mechanisms in the origin of seizures. An important recent advance which is relevant for understanding the cause of epilepsy is the discovery that an excess of excitatory amino acids which act as neurotransmitters can lead to neuronal damage, probably by increasing calcium influx to nerve cells. It appears from recent experimental evidence that neurons with the function to inhibit electrical activity may be the first victims of this toxic effect. In this way, the equilibrium in neuronal networks, where inhibitory feedback loops play an essential stabilizing role, may be disturbed and synchronized oscillations may occur. This is the basic process which leads to seizures. These new findings have prompted investigations with the aim of developing new drugs that can act as antagonists of excitatory amino acids and may be used in order to treat, or even prevent, epileptic disorders.

Nerve Cell Communication and Electrical Signals

Electrical currents in the nervous system are carried by ions which move within the watery solution of the body. In neuronal functions, the most important ion movements occur across cell membranes. All living cells are enclosed by a thin lipid membrane which, in itself, is relatively inpenetrable to watery solutions of ions. The various ions may however, cross the membrane at special sites (probably protein molecules) built into the membrane, called 'ion channels'. In animal cells in general, the intracellular ionic concentrations are drastically different from those of the surrounding fluids. These differences are maintained with the help of so-called 'ion-pumps,' molecules which use metabolic energy for a more or less continuous active transport of ions across the membrane.

For communication purposes nerve cells thus make use of 'electrical signals'. The membranes of muscle and nerve fibers contain particular ion channels which open or close depending on the amount of electrical potential difference across the cell membrane. Through complex interacting processes an action potential (a transient positive shift of membrane potential) may be produced by a change in membrance potential, and this will act as an electrical stimulus for neighboring membrane areas (cf. the progressive 'falling wave' of a row of domino-bricks). Hence, the action potential will progressively propagate along the cell membrane until the end of the nerve fiber has been reached.

Branches of nerve fibers normally terminate close to the membrane of other nerve cells. The two adjecent membranes do not fuse, but remain separated by a small distance of about 20-50nm, called the synaptic cleft. Across this distance, communication between the two cells is usually mediated by particular chemical messengers. These chemical messengers are released by nerve endings when they are invaded by an action potential. Once a chemical messenger has been released, it diffuses across to the membrane of the next cell. There, the chemical substance (transmitter) influences the post-synaptic cell by combining, briefly, with specific 'receptor' molecules inserted into the membrane. In some cases, the combination of transmitter and receptor leads, more or less directly, to the opening of an ion channel. In such a case, the ion channel may be part of the receptor molecule itself. In other cases, the transmitter-receptor combination leads to a complex series of chemical events (including usage of 'second messengers', such as cyclic AMP) which, ultimately, give rise to a change in the state of ion channels. In the latter case, the channel may be localized at a membrane site separate from that of the receptor molecule.

Each neuron in the central nervous system may be synaptically influenced, more or less simultaneously, by hundreds or thousands of other neurons. Each neuron reacts to the sum of all the excitatory and inhibitory messages that it receives from other cells. Most known neurons react by sending out action potentials along their own axon (an extension of the nerve cell that reaches close to other nerve cells). The intensity of this message is graded by varying the frequency of the action potentials (i.e. their number per unit time). One of the essential functional properties of neurons is their capability to transduce the total intensity of post-synaptic current (i.e. the sum of all the excitatory and inhibitory currents produced by different individual synapses) into a frequency coded signal consisting of a train of repetitive action potentials.

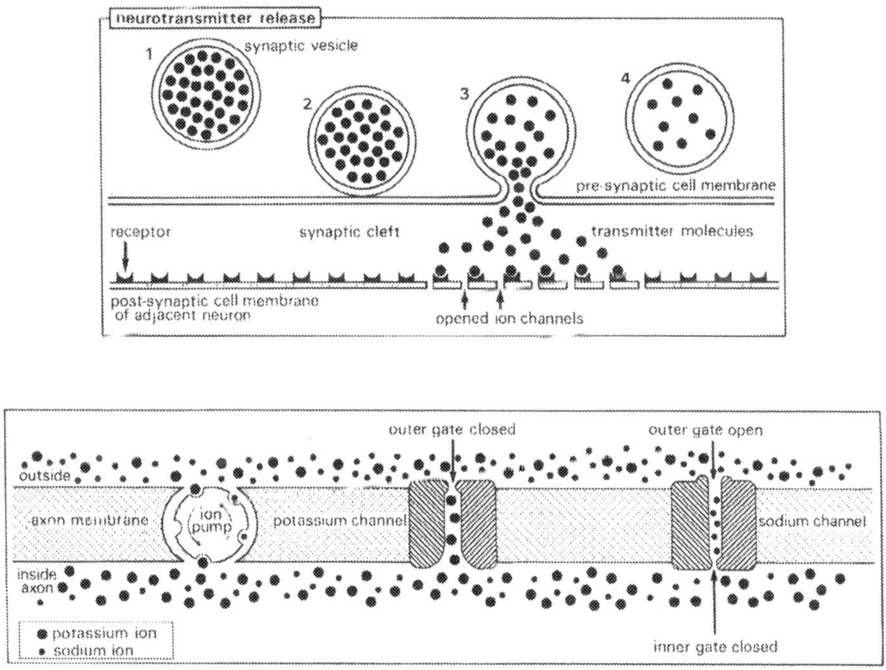

Figure 2 Neurotransmitter Release

Chemical Messengers

The chemical messengers involved in nerve cell communication can be divided into 3 overlapping categories due to their mode of action:

1. neurotransmitters, which act quickly and over short distances to alter transiently the excitability of cells;
2. neuromodulators, which alter the response of a cell to a distinct chemical input;
3. neurohormones, which act at a distance from their site of release and give rise to neuronal effects that tend to be slow in onset.

Disturbances in chemical neurotransmission are involved in a number of neurological and behavioral disorders. The best known example is Parkinson's disease, which is a progressive neurological disorder producing an abnormal slowing of motor sets (movement), tremor, and rigidity. The selective death of certain neurons that use dopamine as a transmitter is responsible for symptoms. This discovery has resulted in attempts to compensate for the deficiencies associated with the disease. In the 1970s, this was realized through development of L-Dopa, a chemical precursor of dopamine, for oral administration as a drug. This treatment has considerably improved the quality of life and also the life-expectancy of those afflicted. One of the major problems at this moment is that L-Dopa after several years of treatment tends to become less effective and produces more side-effects. At the moment new approaches in the treatment of Parkinson's disease are being explored and tested (see Chapter III).

The most diverse group of extracellular chemical messengers are the neuropeptides, which can function as transmitters, modulators or hormones (129).

Neuropeptides

In recent years a large number of neuropeptides have been discovered. Neuropeptides are substances present in nerve cells. It is probably neuropeptides that mediate the extraordinary complicated patterns of communication that take place in the nervous system. Neuropeptides are synthetized in large precursor proteins. These precursors can form different peptides. A cascade of processes lead to the expression of the genetic information into biologically active neuropeptides. These processes control the quantities of neuropeptides synthetized as well as the nature of their biological activity, through size, form, and derivation of the end-product. In this way, sets of neuropeptides with different, opposite, and more selective properties are formed from the same precursor. Neuropeptides are, for example, involved in homeostatic mechanisms in the nervous system. Homeostasis apparently is obtained by the release of antagonistically acting neuropeptides generated from the same precursor. For example, y-MSH, which is part of the precursor peptide pro-opiomelanocortin, functions as an opiate antagonist and is thus able to counteract the opiate-like effects of B-endorphin, which is generated from the same precursor molecule. The precise way in which neuropeptides exert their effects on nervous system functioning remains to be clarified.

It is apparent, however, that neuropeptides modulate many central nervous system effects, ranging from motivation, learning, sexual behavior, and sleep to pain (22). Disturbances at various levels of neuropeptide formation may be underlying causes of nervous system dysfunction. It has been suggested that schizophrenia might be the result of an inborn error in the formation or biological activity of y-endorphin and related peptides in the brain. In some instances y-type endorphins have been shown to have antipsychotic effects in schizophrenic patients. Intra-uterine disturbances, traumatic and infectious disturbances of the brain, and aging may be acquired causes of psychiatric and neurological disease in which the formation of neuropeptides is disturbed and is responsible for part of the symptoms. For example, the treatment of mild memory disturbances resulting from brain trauma with vasopressin neuropeptides appears to be beneficial. Furthermore, ACTH neuropeptides have in some cases been shown to have effects on cognition and mood in mildly disturbed elderly people. In animal experiments on nerve cell regeneration, these neuropeptides show promising results.

Much more work is needed to determine the exact influence of the numerous neuropeptides in nervous system functioning. The results with neuropeptides in the clinic so far have been less dramatic than developments in the laboratory. One of the main problems is the mode of administration of neuropeptides, which do not penetrate in sufficient amounts through the blood-brain-barrier.

However, animal experiments suggest that mere picogram amounts, injected directly into the brain, are adequate to achieve effects, and such amounts are difficult to measure in the brain. Neuropeptides may have dual or complex effects, and may elicit different responses following acute or chronic administration. Because of these effects, it can be difficult to determine dose, frequency and duration of treatment. Many of these problems might be solved if more sensitive methods for detection and measurement of neuropeptides in body fluids and the brain become available. Monoclonal antibodies and short-lived isotopes that can be used as markers, combined with sophisticated imaging devices, are already available for these purposes. More knowledge on the bioavailability, kinetics, and lipid solubility is needed to improve treatment. Knowledge on the structural requirements of neuropeptide-receptor interaction is needed in order to enable the synthesis of analogues and of conventional compounds which are more rigid ;and as such they may be more effective than the original endogenous ligands. Ligands are the substances with which cell receptors interact selectively to bring about biological effects.

In the coming decades, many more biologically active peptides will certainly be discovered. In the future it may be expected that the present drugs for the treatment of psychopathological disorders will be replaced by neuropeptides, neuropeptide analogues, and eventually their more rigid imitations with more specific and less side effects than the drugs in use today. This will lead to a more fundamental approach to the treatment of psychiatric and neurological diseases, retardation, aging, and possibly dementia.

Interactions of the Nervous and Immune Systems and the Environment

As mentioned above, nervous system disorders involve disturbances in the dynamic interaction between central nervous system, the rest of the organism, and its environment. A health-related issue that illustrates this fact is the phenomenon of stress and the biological response it elicits in the form of a complex interaction between the nervous system and the immune system.

Scientific interest in the relevance of stress to health and disease developed early this century. For example, Walter Cannon, Hans Selye, and John Mason discovered that animals exposed to serious physical or psychological conditions exhibited a number of hormonal and physiological responces (41). Recent multidisciplinary research has led to a renaissance of the interest in stress and its role in health and disease. According to current thinking, stress is a general (but not completely unspecific) response of the brain and the rest of the body to environmental factors. Environmental factors or conditions that affect the organism are often called 'stressors'. How animal and man respond to such stressors depends on individual psychological and physiological characteristics. This complex interaction determines, then, why one person would suffer under certain stressor conditions while the other remains healthy, why one person acquires an immune disease while the other gets a coronary infarction. In general, unpredictable stressors in an uncontrollable environment represent the greatest hazard for health both in animal and man (41).

Within the body, three complex subsystems - the nervous, endocrine, and immune systems interact to regulate the adaptive response of the individual to stressors. This interaction is multilateral. The brain controls bodily functions via neuroendocrine and autonomic mechanisms. The immune system is also influenced by neural and neuroendocrine mechanisms originating in the brain. For example, direct effects of the autonomic nervous system on lymphoid tissues such as thymus and milt has been demonstrated in animals (42). Changes in the concentration of certain neuroactive compounds, such as VIP, enkephaline and noradrenaline, may affect functioning in the various lymphoid tissues. Prolactin, vasopressin, ACTH and various other neuropeptides have been shown to affect lymphocyte function (10).

Conversely, it has been demonstrated that lymphoid tissue is able to produce some of the same chemical messengers as those produced in the nervous system (13). These have been shown to affect the function of the nervous system during an ongoing immune response. This area is of great interest, as many neurological and behavioral diseases are associated with responses of the immune system.

Myasthenia gravis is an interesting example of a disease that involves both the immune and the nervous system. Myasthenia gravis is a progressive, muscle-paralyzing disease resulting from the body's destruction of receptor sites on muscles that bind the neurotransmitter acetylcholine. Acetylcholine controls muscle contraction. The 'autoimmune attack' causes serious muscle weakness. Myasthenia gravis is now being treated with procedures that decrease the immune response and with drugs that increase the nerve to muscle communication (5).

Multiple sclerosis (MS), as mentioned above, seems to be another disease involving both the nervous and the immune system. The immune attack in MS may be against a component of the fatty myelin sheath around nerves (5). The autoimmune hypothesis has been strengthened by the discovery of an association between certain human leukocyte antigen (HLA) types and the disease (104).

Substance Use Disorders

During the last decades a marked increase in the use of alcohol, legal and illicit psychoactive drugs has been seen in most industrialized countries. The percentage of the population in the Netherlands with problems related to addictive substances, for example, may approach 10 percent in the near future. Addiction presents a complex pattern of interacting social, psychological, and biological factors. Behavioral medicine may lead to further understanding of addiction; basic neuroscience may contribute to understanding the biology underlying addiction (99).

This chapter considers some endogenous factors involved in drug dependence. In recent years, progress has been made by the discovery and analysis of the so-called 'pleasure-centers' in the brain and the possible involvement of neuropeptides in drug self-administration. When electrodes are placed in the pleasure centers, animals readily learn, for example, to press a lever to obtain electrical stimulation of such brain sites. These brain stimulation reward centers are probably the sites where addictive drugs elicit self-administering behavior. Interestingly, changes in the threshold for brain stimulation reward seem to reflect changes in mood. Neuropeptides and hormones modulate many central nervous system processes. They seem also to be concerned in reward mechanisms and drug self-administration. Animals self-administer endogenous morphine-like substances (endorphines). Other neuropeptides, such as those related to vasopressin, influence heroin self-adminstration in animals. Thus, these and other neuropeptides may contribute to individual susceptibility in animals for the development of addiction. In this respect, increased knowledge may permit identification of individual variations in biological susceptibility to certain substances. It is also possible that treatment of substance use disorders might improve as a result of a better understanding of addiction. Needless to say, neuroscience research by itself will not solve a complex phenomenon such as the basic mechanisms involved in addiction.

Human research on addiction is hampered, because of the problematic relation between addiction and the medical setting, including clinical research, and the almost lack of instruments to investigate addictive behavior in detail. Since recently substance use disorders have been identified as mental disease entities, it might well be that interest in human addiction research can be stimulated. This should include the discription of the disease in relation to other mental disorders like depression and schizophrenia, the commonalities and differences between addiction to various drugs and habits, the personality of the addicts, the application of sophisticated psychometric test procedures in order to search for abnormalities in information processing, clinical trials for evaluating therapeutic interventions and the analysis of physiological processes in the body in relation to drug seeking behavior.

Pain

Another case where the interaction of somatic, mental and social factors is of importance is in chronic pain. There are two major types of chronic pain: one is due to some form of malignancy, and the other is the so-called 'chronic benign pain syndrome,' in which complaints of the skeletomotor system and headaches predominate. Three main methods of alleviating pain are usually advocated: drugs, instrumental techniques, and psychotherapeutic or behavioral approaches. One of the important discoveries in recent years was the identification of endogenous (present in the body), morphine- like substances called endorphines that act at specific receptors in the brain and spinal cord and modulate sensitivity and emotional response to painful stimuli.

Narcotic (centrally acting) analgesics (drugs for pain) act on specific 'opiate receptors' in the CNS, which are in fact receptors for the neurotransmitters enkephalin or endorphin. The discovery of the endorphins as the endogenous ligands (36) for these opiate receptors has been a major breakthrough in the understanding of pain and pain suppression by the organism itself, and of the mechanism of action of narcotic analgesics. The hope that powerful analgesics might be developed without the detrimental side effects of tolerance and addiction, however, has so far not been realized.

One new and helpful technique for some people with chronic malignant pain is to apply morphine locally in the dorsal part of the spinal cord by epidural catheter.

With regard to purely instrumental techniques, transcutaneous electrical nerve stimulation, stimulation of central brain structures, acupuncture, and interruption of afferent (going into the brain) pathways by peripheral nerve blocks have been, and still are, applied. A promising new technique is vascular decompression of cranial nerves in some forms of neuralgias, e.g., in the trigeminal nerve.

Pain, however, is not only a personal sensory experience (nociception). It also comprises affective, behavioral, and cognitive components that may lead to observable behaviors. Such pain-elicited behavior may be positively reinforced by sympathetic reactions from the environment, in accordance with the mechanisms of operant conditioning. In the early 1960s, behavioral methods were introduced in pain treatment programs, not to cure pain, but rather to treat excess disability and expressions of suffering in chronic benign pain (e.g., low-back pain). Based on these principles, many kinds of comprehensive pain management programs have been developed, with an emphasis on coping with pain, rather than on pain relief.

Affective Disorders

Another example of the importance of dynamic interactions between the internal and external milieus and the interplay between events at the levels of behavior and somatic functions is found in affective disorders. Affective disorders are among the most common psychiatric disorders. Ten, perhaps 20 percent of the population, will experience disabling depression at some time of life; about 0.5 percent of people suffer from mania, frequently in combination with depression.

The expanding interest in the somatic aspects of affective disorders has been stimulated by observations of the therapeutic effectiveness of somatic interventions, such as the administration of antidepressants and lithium, electroconvulsive treatment (ECT), and the manipulation of sleep. The effectiveness of psychotropic drugs and ECT has inspired investigators to put forward an increasing number of biochemical hypotheses to explain these effects and the pathophysiology of the affective disorders. In particular, disturbances in the transmission of information between cells in the nervous system have been considered (14). Because chemical processes in the human brain are at present inaccessible to direct measurement before death, there is a need for techniques that can observe chemical changes in various parts of the brain (see brief on new diagnostic techniques later in this Chapter). Biological psychiatrists are now investigating hormonal processes supposedly reflecting chemical brain mechanisms. They also use blood cells as models for studying biochemical events in the brain. Chemical studies of human brain tissue in various disorders after death have become increasingly frequent.

The antidepressant effects of sleep manipulations represent another source of theorizing on the background of affective disorders (60). Especially hypotheses on the critical role of disturbed chronobiological mechanisms regulating arousal, activation and sleep have inspired much therapeutic and fundamental research in this area.

These strategies have led to an enormous accumulation of knowledge, but insights into the specific causation and treatability of affected disorders remain limited. Any approach will remain insufficient as long as one considers events on the levels of experience and behavior as mere consequences of a somatic disorder, rather than as essential processes relating to the interactions of the total organism with the environment. The result of this view is that the attention is predominantly directed to the physical level of functioning. Only the study of interreactions between events on the levels of experience, behavior, and somatic functions rather than the somatic functions per se will elucidate the contribution of the latter to the causation of affective disorders and the role of somatic prevention or treatment methods.

Future progress will come from a more integrative approach. The affective disorders result from dynamic interactions between the internal and external milieus. Disturbed patterns of experience and behavior in the individual must certainly receive the same attention as do physical disturbances. The links between somatic models and sociological, psychological, or behavioral models are week and should be strengthened. More integrated research combining different disciplinary points of view is needed. The main advances should be made by multidisciplinary research teams, in which experts in the behavioral and neurosciences jointly study patients, healthy subjects and animals, each providing their own expertise for the analysis of phenomena on all levels of behavioral and somatic organization.

Neuropsychology

Development of new techniques in neuropsychology, the science which relates psychological processes to the underlying biological processes has extended the range of possibilities for examining cognitive and other higher functions in people (82). The various techniques which are being used include the following (68):

- qualitative analyses, with the help of procedures derived from behavioral neurology, in which basic motor functions and auditory, tactile, and visual modalities are investigated.
- psychometric approaches, in which various cognitive functions are assessed with the help of standard and normalized psychological tests, such as intelligence scales. This psychometric test-tradition is particularly strong in the clinical setting.
- approaches based on information processing paradigms are being developed with the aid of computer methods. Psychological and cognitive processes are examined by analyzing behavior in terms of quantifiable components and qualitative patterns.

Ultimately, it may be the combination of these procedures that is optimal in yielding a behavioral description of psychological functions and dysfunctions in individuals (69).

Psychological techniques are used to assess the state of patients with neurological and psychiatric diseases as well as the effects of the aging process, and the effects of interventions (drug treatment, environmental changes, etc.). A number of neurological diseases, including Alzheimer's disease and Parkinson's disease, as well as certain forms of brain injury, manifest themselves at a behavioral level (69; 70). An extensive neuropsychological examination of the individual subject may thus enable early diagnosis of the disease. In general, a description of the cognitive and behavioral status may lead to a better understanding of the nature of the processes involved and may guide intervention techniques based upon pharmacotherapy and environmental manipulation. These techniques are also useful in the evaluation of the behavioral, affective, and cognitive implications of psychoactive drugs and side-effects of conventional medication, such as neuroleptics, antidepressants, minor tranquilizers, and hypnotics.

An issue of growing importance in applied neuropsychology is education. A better understanding of the neuropsychology of, for example, learning, memory, the reading process, and attention may be used in designing education programs for both normal and disabled children and adults. The successful adaptation of people to their environment is obviously critically dependent on learning. Individuals who are deficient in basic learning skills are especially handicapped in coping with the complexities of modern society (29).

Mechanisms of learning are studied at various levels of the central nervous system. In the next Chapter the role of neuronal plasticity in learning will be discussed.

One of the remarkable characteristics of the human brain is the specialization of the left and right cortical hemispheres for different cognitive, perceptual, and language functions. Much research interest is directed towards understanding the specialization of the left and right hemisphere in perceptual strategies and the relation of language processes to particular zones of the left hemisphere of the brain (77).

Theories of motor control, attention, lateralisation or the transmission of information between the hemispheres, memory processing, and, in general, human information processing have already broadened perspectives on neuropsychological assessment, and probably will continue to do so in the future. A point of considerable importance refers to the introduction of microcomputer-based technology in clinical settings. Computer-assisted expert systems, (psycho)diagnosis and training are especially relevant in this respect. Future research interests will probably be directed to the role of sub-cortical (e.g. limbic system) structures in the organization and expression of emotions. Another field of interest will be in the interface between the hypothalamic-pituitary structures and the regulatory mechanisms of behavior. The relationship between pharmacological parameters and psychological processes remains an area of specific interest. In the future neurochemistry and molecular biology will contribute to neuropsychological insights. The relation between neurotransmission or neurohumoral activity and behavior is considered to be of special importance in this respect. Research is also investigating endocrinological variables such as pituitary hormones, related neuropeptides, and their corresponding neuronal systems in relation to memory disorders and potential effects on cognitive processes.

Information Technology, Prosthetics and Diagnostics

The rapid pace of advance in the fields of micro-electronics, materials science, bio-engineering, and knowledge of nerve and muscle control, will result in far more sophisticated neurological prosthetics. Neurological prostheses are defined as wholly or partly implanted devices which stimulate nerve fibres or nerve cells electrically and thereby restore functions of the nervous system that have been lost as a result of disease or injury.

In the area of communicative disorders, a number of new and future prosthetics can be anticipated. Implantable or portable sensory aids for hearing, speech, vision, and even smell may be developed. These will result from gaining the ability to electrically stimulate individual sensory nerves, selective parts of the spinal cord, and areas on the surface or within the brain. Coupled with these abilities will be concomitant progress in microprocessor developments, as well as advances in the theories of signal processing, to emulate sight and hearing.

Speech control devices will use computer-generated speech which will be directly controlled by the central nervous system. In the area of vision, new developments involve visual devices which use direct cortical stimulation. Visual signal eye prosthetics and the possibility of the artificial eye will, however, need a real breakthrough to become viable.

The area of human movement is another area with a high future technological potential. One of the advances is directed towards movement control systems, which use signals from peripheral nerves and/or spinal roots to control artificial limbs in amputees. Furthermore, the continuous advances with new lighter and more durable materials will improve the problem of interfacing prosthetic devices with the patient's skin.

In addition, attempts to use electromechanical and electronic devices to aid in the functioning of damaged nerves should be taken into account. A promising technology in this area is functional electrical stimulation. This technique is based on the utilization of electrical activation of uninnervated (lacking nerve stimulation) skeletal muscle as a means of affecting movement (127). The primary goal is to provide useful movement of the upper and lower extremities in persons with paralysis due to trauma or disease. Its use as a long-term assistive aid (orthosis) in paralysis has yet to reach the stage of clinical applications. This is due to a number of factors, including:

1. Implant devices rather then surface stimulators will be required for long term use. Such devices will require many channels in order to stimulate a large number of muscle groups and incorporate advanced microprocessor technology to permit setting and control

of many parameters and signals. Both the biomaterial and electronic design problems are great, but fast moving advances in technology suggest that these problems will be solved in 4 to 6 years.

2. Electrodes that exist today are associated with many problems. It is still not clear whether the muscle or the peripheral nerve should be stimulated and with what form of electrode this should be done. Present research promises to resolve these questions within a few years.

3. Control systems that duplicate the complex function of the neuromuscular system have yet to be perfected. Their design requires an understanding of how the normal body is able to position the extremities, maintain balance, and control timing and force. Again, present research has produced many useful results and should provide the basis for clinically useful devices in 4 to 6 years, but these systems will be rudimentary and it will be many years before the more sophisticated human activities like running or dancing could even be contemplated.

An important spin-off of the recent developments in information technology concerns the area of brain imaging and diagnosis. The central, and to a lesser extent the peripheral nervous system, are highly inaccessible to direct investigation of physiological functions and disease processes. The introduction of new non-invasive imaging techniques, such as positron emission tomography (PET), and magnetic resonance imaging (MRI), along with magnetoencephalography (MEG), and computerized electroencephalography (EEG), is rapidly changing this situation (17).

New Diagnostic Techniques

PET scanning belongs to the realm of nuclear medicine. PET scanning uses radioactive isotopes (with a short half-life) of elements such as oxygen, carbon, fluorine and nitrogen. These radioisotopes are used to label selected biological compounds that are administered as tracers. The more active brain regions accumulate a tracer and emit radioactive particles (positrons) that can be detected at the scalp. The radiation can be measured by a circular array of detectors outside the body. With the help of a computer, three-dimensional pictures af the brain's ongoing activity can be constructed (75; 103).

PET imaging can provide a noninvasive, regional assessment of many biochemical processes that are essential to the normal functioning of the organ that is being visualized (123). PET thus has capabilities that go beyond those of any existing diagnostic technique. It provides functional information, while other types of imaging (such as CT or CAT scans) give only anatomical information (100).

The advantage of PET scanning is that the radioactive materials used have a very short half-life time. That means that radioactivity disappears from the body of the patient rather quickly after the procedure. However, such materials can only be made by a cyclotron. It is also necessary to have at the site where the measurements are to be carried out a rather sophisticated radiochemical laboratory to prepare the materials for injection

Magnetic resonance imaging (MRI) is based on the magnetic properties of atomic nuclei. Hydrogen atoms in biological tissue have a polarity (that is, they have a magnetism). When placed in a magnetic field, they align themselves with the field. A radio frequency can then be applied at right angles to the main field, which causes the atoms to precess (or 'wobble') in phase. When the radio field has been turned off, the nuclei continue to precess in phase, generating a similar radio frequency. This can be picked up by receiver coils as the atoms return to their normal position. These signals can be used to construct images, using mathematical analysis and reconstruction done by computer.

A three-dimensional projection of the distribution of hydrogen in the body clearly shows the division into different tissues. This is especially useful in the distinction of soft tissues, e.g., the white and grey matter of the brain (30). In MRI a spatial resolution below 0.5mm will soon be reached, which implies that delicate neuropathological alterations can be detected (23).

The significance of **magnetic resonance spectroscopy** (MRS) lies in its potential ability to give insight into a number of the body's metabolic processes, for example, on the concentration of metabolites, pH in the cell, metabolism of labelled compounds, the kinetics of enzymatic reactions, and the concentration of ions in the body. This information may eventually be used to distinguish between normal and abnormal cells. A combination of MRS and MRI in one unit seems technically feasible (58; 102).

Magnetoencephalography (MEG). MEG is a new brain imaging technology that assesses brain function by measuring the very subtle magnetic fields generated inside the scalp by nerve cell activity. It precisely measures and locates minute changes in magnetic fields, generated by

the flow of ionic currents (electricity) through nerve fibers. No ionizing radiation, radioactive isotopes, or strong man-made magnetic fields are needed to produce MEG pictures of the brain.

Sensory stimuli produce patterns of activity in the sensory pathways and cerebral cortex that can be measured in the form of small voltage changes (evoked potentials) in the scalp by electroencephalogram (EEG). New diagnostic tests of sensory and neurological disorders have been developed using evoked potentials. MEG, combined with the EEG, makes it possible to localize active populations of neurons more precisely than with electrical recordings alone. For this purpose, special packages of programs based on advanced mathematical techniques are being developed.

New imaging techniques can be used to visualize the metabolic and electrical activity in the human brain. New in modern imaging techniques is the measurement of processes in time, cf., the introduction of motion pictures in the world of photography. The visualization of regional blood flow, glucose (sugar) utilization, and the labelling of drugs may provide information on the brain's energy metabolism and the kinetics of drug use by the central nervous system. With PET, for instance, tracer amounts of drugs, analogues of drugs, or endogenous constituents are used to monitor either a biochemical conversion (e.g. glucose metabolism or protein synthesis) or to label a particular molecule (e.g. ligands for receptors or enzymes). These techniques are of great importance as research tools. They also have significant clinical applications, which will probably increase (116).

Imaging techniques will enable the early diagnosis and the estimation of the extent and irreversibility of brain infarcts, transient ischemic attacks, and tumors. The diagnosis of neurodegenerative diseases, such as Parkinson's disease, Huntington's disease, or Alzheimer's disease is highly facilitated by modern imaging techniques (see Chapter III). In the case of many psychiatric diseases, the precise brain pathology is still not understood. Modern imaging may help determine, for instance, whether subtle changes in brain tissue exist in certain classes of schizophrenia (there is no consensus on the existence of brain tissue pathology in such cases) (20).

In the diagnosis of epilepsy, the EEG recording and transmission technology based on miniaturized electronic devices make it possible to perform long-term EEG monitoring. This is very useful in the diagnosis of certain forms of epilepsy, since the likelihood of detecting seizures is increased. The possibilities of MEG in localizing foci that can initiate a seizure are being investigated. PET may, for instance, distinguish between generalized or focal epilepsy on the basis of glucose utilization (using labelled deoxyglucose).

The combined use of the mapping techniques, together with precise behavioral measurements may lead to new advances in understanding the brain. In the years to come it will be increasingly necessary, however, to compare the costs and benefits of the combined use of the many imaging devices available.

In summary, the examples of progress in neurosciences research presented in this chapter illustrate the high scientific and technological potential of the field. To fulfill its promises for future health benefits, however, integration of the monodisciplinary approaches into multidisciplinary programs is needed. Adequate financial, human, and technological resources are required.

Scientific and technological progress in the neurosciences will raise new public policy issues in the years to come. New technologies for prevention and treatment may, for example, affect health services planning as dramatically as did the introduction of neuroleptic (tranquilizer) drugs in the 1950s. Advances in brain imaging mandate a careful comparison of the costs and benefits of the combined use of the several imaging devices available. The use of genetic markers introduces complex ethical questions.

In the next chapters, such implications will be systematically analyzed with regard to one specific case study: the regeneration, repair, and reorganization of nervous tissue.

Chapter II – The Reorganization, Regeneration, and Repair of Nervous Tissue

Recovery of function in people after damage to the brain or spinal cord was considered out of question for many years. It was generally believed that severed neurons in adults did not regrow and that no functionally significant structural adjustments could occur in the central nervous system. In contrast, peripheral nerves were known to regenerate after being injured (51). The axons (threadlike extensions of nerve cells along which information travels) of peripheral nerves can regrow after being damaged, leading to a slow return of feeling and movement after certain injuries.

Recent observations, however, suggest that the central nervous system also has considerable ability to adapt to damage either by compensatory mechanisms or by local tissue regeneration. The nervous system thus is not a static network of cells merely arranging communication between organs within an organism or between the organism and its environment. The nervous system is now seen to be of a much more dynamic nature, which may change in response to altered conditions inside or outside the organism. The ability of the nervous system to change its activity as a result of previous experience or in response to injury is called **neural plasticity**.

Nervous system plasticity encompasses a breadth of phenomena. It can involve the molecular level, for example, changes in neuronal membranes. It can also involve the behavioral level, for example, with changes in behavior to cope with a changing environment. Thus, neural plasticity is an essential and central feature of adaptation. It includes normal adaptive processes, such as the development of the brain and the modification of neurons on the basis of experience. It also includes the response to abnormal events such as brain and spinal cord injury, toxins, and malnutrition. Nervous system plasticity is of importance in relation to a number of important health-related problems, such as brain injury, developmental disorders, learning disabilities, and dementia.

This Chapter will present findings in different areas of plasticity research. Subsequently, it will briefly discuss potential technological developments based on these findings, including transplantation, drugs, and environmental interventions.

Development of Basic Circuits in the Brain

The circuitry of the brain is determined, in the first instance, by genetic factors. However, it is becoming increasingly clear that genetic information is not sufficient to specify the large number of synaptic connections in the brain, which in a mammal may amount to 10^{15}. Although genes determine overall aspects of brain architecture and wiring patterns, non-genetic factors can modify this basic organization (6). These factors are internal or external in nature. Among the former, hormones are very important. Among the latter are included nutrition, sensory and motor experience, learning, and social interactions. Extragenetic factors seem to exert their greatest influence early in development, although they can also modify synaptic connections in the adult brain. This section will examine a few of these extragenetic factors.

The role of hormones is best illustrated by the fact that during development the sexual hormones have a strong influence on the differentiation not only of body organs but also of the brain. Sexual hormones are responsible for the organization of specific circuits in the brain of the developing animal. In general, it can be said that the developing brain of an animal of either genetically determined sex has the potential to differentiate either in a female or a male direction. The human brain is differentiated sexually, and the presence of sex hormones during development may permanently determine human behavior.

Another example of the influence of hormones on the nervous system is provided by bird song. Songs of passarine birds are learned during a critical period of their early life. In this phase, they must hear the song in order to learn the acoustic pattern. In some species, singing is restricted to males. The capacity to sing depends on circulating androgens (male hormones), and fluctuates with the seasons. An important advance in understanding the underlying processes was the discovery by Nottebohm (1981) that singing in these birds depends on a number of specialized areas of the brain (98). During the critical period for singing, sex steroids determine the number and even the structure of the neurons in the 'song areas' of the brain. Under the influence of androgens the neurons of these areas show growth of their dendrites (hair-like protrusions of the nerve cell) and reorganization of their synapses. Experiments indicate that giving testosterone (male sex hormone) or cholesterol to adult birds promotes such changes, but it is not yet clear how this relates to behavioral plasticity.

In the hypothalamus a similar system, showing reversible synaptic formation in response to a changing need for hormones, can be found. Under conditions indicating that more of a hormone is needed, reversible morphological (physical) changes of specific nuclei can be observed. It appears that by these changes synchronized firing of the neurons is promoted, facilitating release of the hormones. This is a form of synaptic plasticity which serves clear physiological functions.

An important external factor which affects development is the experiences to which an animal is exposed in early stages of development. A well-known example is the acquisition of a particular behavior during a critical period of life which has been called imprinting by Lorentz (85). For example, Lorentz studied what occurs when a duck, in an early phase of development, is exposed to a moving object. The duck learns to follow that object. This is the phenomenon of imprinting. Of course, under normal circumstances the moving object will be the mother duck.

How early experience influences the development of the brain has been particularly well-established as regards the visual system (see brief).

The interface between the nervous system and the muscles also show plastic changes under the influence of use. In mammals the pattern of activation of muscles appears to play an important role in the formation of muscle contractile properties. Furthermore, increased activity leads to increased levels of the enzymes responsible for the transmission of impulses from the nerve to the muscle. When these synapses are not used, the levels of these enzymes decrease.

There is a growing body of evidence showing that the number and structure of synapses in the brain is dependent on specific environmental factors as exemplified below in the visual system. An important question is whether the intensity of social interactions provided by an enriched environment can have a general influence on structure and function. There are clear indications that rats reared in an enriched environment have cortical neurons showing more extensive branching of their dendrites than similar rats reared in isolation. These neurons, then, have a larger number of connections. However, the effects of enriched environments for humans needs further investigation.

The human and animal nervous systems show plastic properties. These depend not only on genetic and hormonal factors, but also on the intensity of sensory and motor messages that pass through the nervous system. Furthermore, the general environment in which a human or an animal grows up plays an important role in shaping its brain.

This ability to modify brain circuitry in response to a changing environment is essential to human adaptation and survival. Present-day industrial society, with its exposures to drugs, toxins, or radiation, could affect synaptic connections and brain chemistry adversely and thus lead to disorders in functioning. This is particularly true during early development (59).

Early Experience and Brain Development

A cat or a monkey deprived of visual information by suturing the eyelids of one eye during a critical period will be unable to see with the deprived eye even after the sutures are removed. This effect is only observed during a defined period, varying between species, occuring in early development. An important observation is that visual deprivation causes physiological and physical changes in the visual cortex of the brain. Indeed, after closure on one eye the columns of cells of the visual cortex which normally receive signals from that eye shrink and the columns corresponding to the other eye expand. It is interesting to note that the effect of the closure of both eyes is much less pronounced. This indicates that the changes which occur in the visual cortex of the one-eye deprived animal are due to an unbalance between the impulses reaching the cortex from both eyes. Furthermore, it has been shown by Hubel and Wiesel (1970) that in an animal which squints, no cells can be found in the visual cortex which respond to stimulation of both eyes simultaneously (66). Thus, it appears that in the normal animal the nerve fibres reaching the visual cortex from both eyes share a common neuronal network. However, during development they compete for the space in the brain. The experimental findings described here are not only of interest in understanding the development and organization of the visual cortex, but they also indicate that similar changes in brain organization may occur in other systems if the normal inputs are not activated at a given time.

Factors promoting neuron survival and growth

Since the middle of this century, it has been evident that different substances can regulate growth in the nervous system. It is now increasingly clear that neurotrophic factors i.e., factors that are responsible for neuronal survival and growth not only are effective in the development of the nervous system, but continue to play an important role in the adult nervous system, both during physiological conditions and after cell damage.

Presently, several families of factors can be distinguished. One type is the neurotrophic or 'nourishing' factors (NTFs), e.g., nerve growth factor. These factors are involved in neuronal development, survival, and death. They may be supplied by the target area. In addition to these general growth factors, there are neurite-promoting factors (NPFs) that enhance the outgrowth of neuronal processes from the cell body. In addition to the NTF's and the NPF's, which may act directly and generally from the environment surrounding a neuron, there are factors that are mostly bound on cell surfaces and that are involved in guidance of the directional orientation of growing processes from neurons (neurites) (128).

The capacity of the peripheral and central nervous systems to regenerate differ. Studies of sensory neurons, which have both a central and a peripheral fiber, suggest that glial cells (neuron-supporting cells of the CNS) influence this regenerative capacity. Glial cells that surround the axons can myelinate them (cause them to be enveloped in a fatty insulating material). Peripheral nerves are myelinated by Schwann cells; in the brain and spinal cord, the myelinating cells are oligodendrocytes. This means that the interaction between Schwann cells and neurons in the periphery is different from that of oligodendrocytes and neurons in the central nervous system. Schwann cells play an active role in neuronal repair mechanisms. Research findings show that Schwann cells produce proteins such as laminin that have been found to promote the growth of axons and their adhesion to a surface (111). Schwann cells may also produce nerve growth factor. These findings open up possibilities to use peripheral glia to support regeneration of damaged fibers in the central nervous system. For example, in spinal cord injuries, bridges of peripheral nerve grafts could be used.

The best studied neurotrophic factor is the nerve growth factor (NGF), first discovered by Levi-Montalcini and Hamburger (1953). Most of the well-documented effects of NGF occur in the peripheral nervous system. Evidence, however, is accumulating that NGF is also beneficial to central nervous system neurons (87). Currently, much research is devoted to the identification, purification, and characterization of neurotrophic factors. The search is facilitated by the introduction of well-defined in vitro model systems, high performance separation procedures, and recombinant DNA technology.

The molecular mechanism of trophic control is still under debate. Several models have been proposed. More research is needed to confirm which explains the observed phenomena.

From the complexity of the connections between neurons, it is evident that the substances which establish and maintain specific cellular associations play a key role in the correct wiring of the neuronal circuits. Furthermore, such molecules are important to proper neuron-glia interaction. One specific class of cell adhesive molecules (CAM) are glycoproteins. Using recombinant DNA techniques, the gene coding for one CAM has been identified (108). Recent research has shown that other cell surface components, such as gangliosides, also play a role in cell survival and growth of neuronal processes. They have been shown to enhance both neuritic growth in vitro and stimulate peripheral nervous system regeneration. They also facilitate behavioral recovery following brain injury in animals (74).

In the last decade it has been shown that neurite growth in the central and peripheral nervous systems during development and after damage is paralleled by an increased expression of specific neuronal growth-associated proteins (GAP) (130). Although their precise function is still unclear, it is assumed that certain of these proteins are involved in communication between the growing neurite and its target (or destination).

From a variety of studies it is evident that the environment of the cell is extremely important for developmental and damage-induced changes in the peripheral and central nervous systems. Experiments have shown that damage to the axon may affect the local balance of regenerative/degenerative influences of either the local production of growth factors or the transport of such factors. More and more, scientists focus on the role trophic factors may play in pathological conditions. The first and most studied condition is the acute damage of the nervous system. However, their role in polyneuropathies, amyotrophic lateral sclerosis (ALS), Parkinson's disease, and

Alzheimer's disease is being investigated. Likewise, the importance of the defective or deficient supply of trophic factors to normal aging of the peripheral and central nervous systems is currently under study. The assessment of the importance of such factors in the etiology and/or the treatment of diseases can only be performed if appropriate in vivo and in vitro model systems can be developed (3).

In addition to chemical factors that promote cellular growth, cellular membranes are known to generate electric currents that are important for normal cellular development and orientation. A number of studies suggest that regeneration of nervous tissue may be increased by electrical currents, offering possibilities for regenerating peripheral nerves and parts of the spinal cord.

Synaptic Plasticity

Modification of the brain on the basis of experience, learning, or memory is among the most essential manifestations of the plasticity of the nervous system. A matter of great interest for neurobiologists, therefore, are the plastic changes in the nervous system responsible for learning. An important line of research in this respect have been studies of changes in neural networks in relatively simple nervous systems in relation to behavioral changes, for instance in snails (71).

Another line of research is providing evidence that learning can be described in terms of known and specific changes in the synapses of the brain. The long-lasting increase in synaptic transmission is called long-term potentiation (LTP). LTP reflects an important adaptive change in the communication between two neurons and it is even proposed to underlie the mechanism by which newly acquired information in learning processes is stored in neuronal networks. This latter aspect, however, is still under debate.

Physiologically, the phenomenon of LTP is well characterized; a synaptic response may be enhanced for a long period after the application of a series of impulses. This effect can be recorded both in vivo and in vitro. It can be studied in brain slices kept in vitro under conditions which approximate the natural environment of the brain. In particular, a popular preparation used for this purpose is the slice of the hippocampus of the rat, a brain structure which, on the basis of behavioral studies, may play a specialized role in memory. At the cellular level a number of recent observations are starting to shed light on the processes underlying LTP. Two aspects of this problem may be distinguished: one is whether the locus of LTP is pre- or postsynaptic, with evidence both ways. The other aspect of LTP that is currently investigated are the molecular mechanisms that initiate or maintain the adaptive synaptic response (LTP).

One example of research may illustrate the potential of this field. Recently it has been discovered that long-term potentiation depends critically on the activation of NMDA receptors, one of the several types of receptors responding to the neurotransmitter glutamate (28). These NMDA receptors are found in the hippocampus of the brain, and become active only when nerve cells are depolarized. If NMDA receptors are blocked by administering an antagonist, long-term potentiation and learning in a behavioral situation is prevented, suggesting that LTP is involved in some forms of learning (93).

More research at the level of the interaction between biochemical and microphysiological (electrical) properties of the nerve cell processes is urgently needed.

Neural Plasticity and Behavior

The idea is growing in current neuroscience that synaptic plasticity in specific brain regions is related to normal cognitive and other behavioral functions of the brain. This idea is being tested in studies on post-lesion repair mechanisms and recovery of behavioral function, on age-related behavioral deficits and aging of the hippocampus, and on the significance of synaptic potentiation in learning and memory processes. In general, plasticity is the feature of a neuronal circuit that allows adaptation to internal and external stimuli with reference to previous experience. At the behavioral level, plasticity is formulated similarly, emphasizing the adaptive nature of an organism's behavior. In order to cope with a changing environment, an individual should be able to shift from one behavior to another and vice versa. A neural basis for such plasticity is evident from studies of the development of behaviors in close relation to the development of the nervous system; of the organizational and activational effects of hormones on brain and behavior; and of the deterioration of neural and behavioral plasticity in aging organisms.

In animal experiments two approaches have been followed. In the first set of experimental designs, rats are often tested on a single response to a variety of tasks such as maze learning and certain behavioral responses. By comparing the test results of a given test animal in different experimental conditions, one can collect information on the ability to process, acquire, and store new information. In the alternative approach, there are longitudinal studies on fixed motor action patterns or more complex social interactions, which are designed to demonstrate age-related changes in behavioral patterns in a given experimental situation. Together, such studies reveal important information on the adaptive quality of brain and behavior interactions.

If behavioral measurements are to be useful indices of organic disorders, human behavior needs to be described in operational and objective terminology, allowing different types of standardization, including cross-cultural. Such studies should make use of advanced neuro-etiological and neurophysiological test methods. Recently, evidence is accumulating to suggest that such tools may be of relevance to early diagnosis of a variety of brain diseases such as senile dementia of the Alzheimer type and Parkinson's disease. Not only will such approaches aid in the attempt to localize a given disorder to a certain brain region, they will also help to pick up first signs of malfunctioning prior to identification of the disorder by classical medical-biological procedures.

Neural plasticity is now seen as critical in behavioral disorders in which genetic, neurotransmitter, or environmental causes were previously emphasized. Although far from complete, current data suggest that the unique adaptive capability of neuronal circuits is of crucial importance to balance brain and behavioral interactions.

Plasticity research may lead to a number of technological applications. In Chapter III, some applications with regard to Alzheimer's disease, Parkinson's disease, and nervous sytem injury are analyzed.

Transplantation

One potentially important application in the field of neural plasticity is the ability of grafted neurons to partially or wholly replace damaged regions of the brain. It has been shown that embryonic brain tissue can be incorporated both anatomically and functionally into the adult animal central nervous system.

The success of certain transplantation experiments suggests that they might find future clinical application in a number of neuro-degenerative diseases, such as Parkinson's disease and perhaps ultimately Alzheimer's disease (55).

Transplants may be especially promising in the area of peripheral and central nervous system injury. The goal is to restore impaired function below the lesion, usually traumatic. Peripheral nerves can regenerate without intervention, but the direction of the regrowth must be guided. Transplants of peripheral nerves may be more successful through use of materials to support and guide this regrowth. More recent research is directed towards transplants in spinal cord and brain injuries.

Pharmaceutical Developments

A number of natural substances that influence the regeneration of nervous tissue, e.g., neurotrophic factors and gangliosides, have been reviewed. In the future, the production of these substances may be stimulated pharmacologically (124). In addition, drugs similar in structure to some of these factors will probably be developed.

In practice, the design of pharmaceuticals is based on the idea that they should interfere with the dysfunctional processes. Given the plasticity of the brain, however, there is also a need for agents that interact with intact brain regions, possibly involved in compensating for the dysfunction of the damaged brain areas. Positive reactions elicited could counteract the negative symptoms inherent in the disorder.

Environmental Interventions

Earlier sections have discussed the interaction of environmental factors with the development and plasticity of the brain throughout life. Such environmental factors include nutrition, sensory and motor experiences, and social interactions. The importance of the interaction between brain and environment has been demonstrated by environmental deprivation and stimulation experiments in both humans and animals (92). The environment is critical for the development of the newborn and small child. It may also be that environmental interventions have beneficial influences on brain and behavior in later life, especially in the elderly.

Chapter III – Future Technology Approaches and Their Implications for Health

This case study focuses on the **probabilities** of improvements in prevention and treatment of certain nervous system disorders resulting from plasticity research. The potential technological applications of plasticity research include transplantation, pharmaceutical developments, and environmental interventions.

This Chapter analyzes the future applicability of these developments for a number of specific diseases, including Parkinson's disease, Alzheimer's disease, and injury involving nervous system trauma. The choice of these disease categories is based on the anticipated clinical applicability of technological developments in these areas, and on the importance of these conditions in terms of future health needs and health care consequences.

Importance of the Diseases Addressed

Alzheimer's Disease. Alzheimer's disease is one of the most common neurodegenerative disorders. Approximately 7 to 10 percent of the Dutch population 65 years of age and older has some form of dementia (49). Dementia is not a well-defined disease category, but rather a syndrome caused by a number of specific disease entities such as cerebrovascular disorders, brain tumors, infectious diseases, and Alzheimer's disease (94), that can often only be distinguished definitively by postmortem neuropathological examination. Prevalence and incidence figures for dementia differ from country to country, at least partly as a result of inconsistencies in the description of the syndrome and the research methods used. A complicating factor in the Dutch situation is the lack of epidemiological data. Foreign data, pooled from different countries, on the prevalence of 'chronic brain syndrome,' which includes Senile Dementia of the Alzheimer's Type (SDAT) and vascular or arteriosclerotic dementia, have been combined (Table 2).

Using the demographic composition of the Dutch population, the Scenario Report on Aging estimated the number of demented persons (mild cases excluded), based on these prevalence figures (Table 3).

Table 2 Pooled data on the prevalence of chronic brain syndrome

Age	Age- and sex-specific prevalence (percentages)		
	Male (n=1008)	Female (n=1259)	Both sexes (n=2267)
65-69	3.9	0.5	2.1
70-74	4.1	2.7	3.3
75-79	8.0	7.9	8.0
80+	13.2	20.9	17.7
all	6.2	6.3	6.3

Source: (73, pg. 43)

Table 3 Estimates of prevalence of Dementia (mild cases excluded) of the population of 65 years and older in the Netherlands (1983)

Sex	Total number	Percentage
male	44,000	6.4
female	73,000	7.8
male + female	117,000	6.9

Source: (120)

Prevalence and incidence are age-dependent. SDAT accounts for about 50 percent of the irreversible dementia, and is a major cause of death (however, this may not be visible in mortality figures because it is often not registered as the primary cause of death).

Alzheimer's disease is a progressive degenerative disorder of the brain that produces dementia in middle to late life. It is characterized by an ongoing impairment of cognitive functions, personality, and the ability to cope with everyday activities. Late in the course of the disease, many individuals with Alzheimer's become unable to take care of themselves and need full-time care by others. A large fraction of people with Alzheimer's disease are institutionalized, both in nursing homes and hospitals.

While 10 percent of the elderly population are in nursing homes or other geriatric services, as many as 25 percent of demented persons are in such services. Katzman found that in one 500 bed geriatric nursing home in New York, 65 percent of the residents met the clinical and mental status criteria for dementia (72).

Parkinson's Disease. Parkinson's disease is a progressive degenerative disorder that probably starts with the death of certain cells producing the neurotransmitter dopamine. The essential pathology of Parkinson's disease is degeneration of the pigmented neuronal pathways of the brainstem, most evident in the substantia nigra and the locus ceruleus.

The major manifestations of Parkinson's disease are its characteristic tremor, rigidity and inability to initiate voluntary movements. In addition, patients in the late stages of Parkinson's disease may show signs and symptoms of Alzheimer's disease. The motor and cognitive abnormalities accompanying the disease in a more advanced state can make a person a complete invalid and, ultimately, shorten life-expectancy. The estimates of prevalence vary between 60 and 180 per 100,000 in different industrialized countries. The incidence rate is approximately 18 per 100,000 (26). Generally the disease develops, with a gradual onset of symptoms, around 45 years of age. Due to this gradual onset, definitive diagnosis usually does not take place till around 55 years. About 25 percent of the patients survive for 20 years from the onset of the disease. The mortality rate is about 1.6 times higher than in healthy controls (26).

Trauma Involving Nervous Tissue. Brain and spinal cord damage account for a large number of deaths and disabilities each year. Many survivors of severe central nervous system trauma continue to have some form of disability. Since many victims are below 35 years of age, the costs of their care can be enormous. Injury involving peripheral nerves often results in lasting deficits; although peripheral nerves tend to regenerate, functional recovery is often poor.

Brain damage due to accidents results from mechanical force transmitted directly to the underlying brain tissue. Injuries range from transient loss of consciousness, longer periods of unconsciousness, and brain edema, to a greater degree of brain swelling and hemorrhage. Consequences of the latter can include long periods of coma, permanent residual neurological deficits, and posttraumatic epilepsy. Closed head injury can also lead to intracranial hemorrhage, producing hematomas (blood clots). Penetrating head injuries can obviously cause direct damage to the brain. Epidemiological analysis performed in the United States indicate that the rate of head injury is 200 per 100.000 population, with males having approximately a two times higher risk. Age-specific incidence figures show a peak in the 15-24 year old age-group (2; 78; 97). In the Netherlands, an epidemiological study concerning head injury in the area of Groningen, revealed roughly similar trends. Of the 800 to 900 patients admitted to hospitals with head injuries, 18 percent were diagnosed to be serious cases (91).

Traumatic injury of the spinal cord may result in loss of all function below the level of the injury. Estimates of the incidence of traumatic spinal cord injury, based on foreign analyses, find 15 to 30 cases per million persons per year (61; 90; 46). In Dutch hospitals, 450 admissions per year result from spinal cord injuries (119). Studies from other countries indicate that slightly less than half of spinal cord injuries result from traffic accidents.

Those with traumatic spinal cord injury are often young. As a result of intensive medical care, a new patient age 20 has an average remaining life-expectancy of 30 to 40 years (56). The prevalence and demand for care is much larger, therefore, than one may expect on the basis of the relatively low incidence.

Specific epidemiological data on the prevalence and incidence of injury involving peripheral nervous tissue are not available.

Technological Approaches to These Disorders

Transplantation of Nervous Tissue

During the last few years, neural transplantation has been done with increasing frequency, especially in the experimental animal. The medical profession and the public have shown considerable interest in these procedures.

Neural transplantation can be seen primarily as a research tool, advancing the knowledge of the development and repair of the nervous system; it has already resulted in significant gains in knowledge (55; 47; 43). One of the important research contributions of transplant techniques involves trophic or growth promoting factors. Interactions between grafts and the host nervous system has revealed much about their functioning. Trophic factors play a vital role in survival and functioning of the graft. The surgical lesion itself promotes the production of trophic factors. Trophic factors support the survival of cells in the area of the lesion and promote outgrowth. They also may guide the growing axonal tips in the proper direction. In the coming years, transplants will undoubtedly lead to further gains in knowledge. The potential of trophic factors for future pharmacological treatments will be addressed below.

The success of certain transplantation experiments suggests that it might find future clinical application. Clinical applications have been proposed for both the neuro-degenerative diseases and nervous system trauma (12; 55).

One potential clinical application of transplants would be to reverse deficits that result from the loss of certain specific types of neurons. Grafting of neurons, which use monoamines or acetylcholine as their transmitter, is especially important in the context of neurodegenerative diseases. In two neurodegenerative disorders, Parkinson's and Alzheimer's, the progressive and significant loss of such types of neurons probably underlie some of the major clinical symptoms of the disease (11).

In contrast to nervous system injury, where the cause is usually traumatic, the cause of most neuro-degenerative diseases is unknown. It is therefore obvious that the potential significance of transplantation strategies for neuro-degenerative diseases and traumata differ. In clinical terms, one of the major questions is whether neural transplants will affect the underlying disease process in neuro-degenerative diseases.

Parkinson's Disease and Alzheimer's Disease. In Parkinson's disease, damage to neurons producing dopamine in the nigrostriatal system results in a variety of behavioral and motor dysfunctions. Similar dysfunctions have been induced in rats and monkeys by making selective lesions of dopamine producing neurons. The survival and growth of dopamine-rich grafts have been intensively studied in these animal models. The data from rats suggest that grafts of such cells produce new connections to the host brain and spontaneously release sufficient dopamine to correct motor abnormalities. Recently, biomedical scientists have reversed the symptoms of Parkinson's disease in monkeys by successfully transplanting brain cells (105). Such studies on the safety and effectiveness of grafts in monkeys are a critical step towards successful human use.

The progressive loss of memory and other higher mental functions in Alzheimer's disease is associated with neurochemical abnormalities, involving, for example, a loss of acetylcholine in the hippocampus and large parts of the cortex of the brain (37). Interference with cholinergic transmission by cutting the hippocampal fimbria causes severe learning and memory impairments in rats, and thus can be used as an experimental model for some aspects of Alzheimer's. In a number of studies, tissue that supplies the hippocampus with acetylcholine has been transplanted into the cut fimbria or directly into the denervated hippocampus. These studies suggest that such grafts improved these animals' ability to learn a maze. The cerebral cortex is also affected in Alzheimer's disease. It receives its acetylcholine from the nucleus basalis of Meynert (a cluster of cells at the base of the forebrain). These cells degenerate in Alzheimer's. Impairments in this area also result in a decreasing ability of the rat to learn and remember simple tasks. Studies have also suggested that grafts of cells taken from the precursor region of the nucleus basalis of rat embryos and transplanted into the cortex ameliorate their spatial memory (45).

A critical step towards demonstrating the clinical feasibility of neural transplants is to show their safety and effectiveness in non-human primates. Efforts are underway in a number of laboratories to develop such a primate model of Alzheimer's disease.

The first intracerebral neural transplants in humans were performed in Sweden in 1982 and 1983 with a few patients with severe Parkinson's disease (12). In these first clinical applications, tissue from the patient's own adrenal glands was transplanted into the caudate nucleus (part of the brain). These patients had some temporary modest improvement, but overall, results have not been impressive. The major outcome of these procedures was to demonstrate the clinical feasibility of such grafts in humans. Recently, the ethical committee of the University of Lund, Sweden, approved a number of additional transplant procedures with severe Parkinson's disease patients, using human fetal tissue.

If, however, in the future transplantation is to be effective in people with Parkinson's disease a number of issues need to be addressed. One of the issues concerns the to-be-discovered cause of the disease (17). If the causative agent selectively damages neurons producing dopamine, graft tissue may also be susceptible to degeneration and death. In this case, the time period between grafting and degeneration would be a critical factor. If, however, there is a genetic or developmental deficiency in Parkinson's disease that does not affect transplanted dopamine neurons, brain grafting could be an effective therapy in the future. It is also important to know whether the symptoms of dementia that develop late in the course of Parkinson's disease are independent or are secondary to the loss of neurons producing dopamine. If the symptoms are secondary to the loss, brain grafting might be most effective early in the development of the disease.

The future clinical potential for brain grafting in general brain diseases, such as Alzheimer's disease, seems to be limited. The neural degeneration in Parkinson's is much more localized than in Alzheimer's disease. In Alzheimer's disease, the loss of neurons is greater in numbers and the specific neuronal circuitry is not yet known (50). The symptoms observed in the elderly with senile dementia suggest that multiple brain systems are involved in the disease. This poses additional difficulties in determining a site for transplantation.

In both peripheral and central nervous tissue injury the potential clinical application of transplants seems more promising. One of the important reasons is that the lesion is often the result of trauma, and no underlying disease process is involved.

Brain and Spinal Cord Injury. Recent research focuses on enhancing functional recovery after brain injury. Intracerebral transplants might offer promise in the case of certain focal injuries, such as those which occur after penetrating wounds or following surgical removal of a tumor. In laboratory animals, transplanted fetal cells have been sucessfully used to reduce some of the behavioral deficits caused by traumatic injuries. It should be stressed, however, that the degree of behavioral recovery generally is only partial. To date, there is no evidence concerning fetal tissue implants in primates with brain trauma (117).

The ultimate goal of spinal cord transplantation is to restore function below the site of the injury. The strategies used in brain grafting are also applied to the mammalian spinal cord. The following approaches, through which spinal cord function may eventually be recovered, have been used:

1. to implant bridge grafts to permit regeneration of the endogenous fibers (axons of the host spinal cord) and to provide new cells with an increased capacity to generate neuronal processes;
2. to use peripheral nerve transplants **extraspinally** to bridge regions of the cord or between the cord and the brain stem;
3. to implant embryonic central nervous system tissue, which can regenerate into functional spinal cord tissue, in the lesion;
4. To provide the intrinsic circuitry with 'driving' or 'releasing' units.

In the first two approaches, the regeneration of host axons is stimulated through or around the site of injury. Adult peripheral nerve tissue, embryonic tissue, and synthetic materials (such as collagen material) have been used in the first approach to make bridges (106). In general, both in the cases of embryonic and peripheral tissue, it has been shown that the axons can regenerate long distances. A limiting factor, however, is that the regenerative growth ceases when the axons reach the distal (remote) border of the graft. This is also the case when the peripheral nerves are positioned outside the spinal cord. Research is now directed towards constructing an unbroken pathway from the site of the spinal cord injury to the muscle.

Transplanting grafts of peripheral nervous tissue alters the microenvironment surrounding the transected spinal cord. This may also be accomplished by administering chemical preparations (see below) or by the application of electrical energy to the site of the lesion (34). Local electrical stimulation facilitates calcium ion entry at the site of an injured axon and may accelerate axonal outgrowth.

Because of the limited regenerative capacity of damaged spinal cord neurons, the third approach of implanting embryonic central nervous tissue seems promising. It has been shown that embryonic implants can grow axons over long distances in the host spinal cord. If functional synapses are formed within this implant bridge, it is conceivable that a spinal pathway could be restored across the graft.

It is now known that basic elements of locomotion consist of groups of neurons in the spinal cord. These so-called 'locomotion generators' interact in a complex way with neurons whose axons descend from the brain stem and release catecholamine neurotransmitters. Recently, it has been suggested that paralysis caused by spinal cord injury might respond to grafts of embryonic catecholamine neurons into the spinal cord near the locomotion generators, even if the spinal pathways are not repaired (46). Considering the influence of monoamines on spinal cord function, this model promises possibilities of analyzing the functional specificity of these implants. This could be an important step towards using implants in the clinical setting.

Peripheral Nerve Repair. Injury to peripheral nerves, such as those in the arms and hands often results in lasting motor and sensory deficits. Peripheral nerves have a larger capacity to regenerate and reach their peripheral targets than nerve cells within the central nervous system (21). This process can be affected positively. However, recovery of function is still often poor. One of the crucial elements of functional recovery seems to be the accuracy of the patterns of regeneration. To date, clinicians have manipulated regenerating neurites both physically and chemically to improve functional outcome.

Surgical repair of lesions of peripheral nerves has been attempted for decades. Both biological and non-biological tissues have been used to bridge nerve defects. In clinical practice, nerve grafts are used when suturing of the nerve is not possible because the gap is too large. Good clinical functional results using autologous (derived from the same individual) nerve grafting techniques have been obtained. Small nerve allografts have been reported to survive and function occasionally, in both experimental and clinical studies (113). Ideally, nerve grafts shoud be easily accepted by the host without producing any significant side effects. Matching for major histocompatibility antigens improves the survival and functional recovery of nerve allografts (113).

Another approach to stimulate regeneration of nerve fibers involves artificial substances. Nerve gaps have been closed by using a bridging tube, fitted onto the two nerve ends. Results are disappointing. Recently, researchers have developed an artificial template to guide the regrowth of regenerating nerves. The template consists of a cross-linked collagen matrix and is similar to materials used to encourage skin regrowth. Severed sciatic nerves linked by the collagen guide grew together across gaps as wide as 3/4 inch in laboratory rats. This is the first instance of nerve regrowth without the use of supplemental nerve tissue (88).

Pharmacological Developments
Plasticity research opens possibilities for new pharmacological developments. Research findings have shown that several families of trophic factors exist, regulating growth and cell survival in the nervous system (128). On the basis of this knowledge, two major pharmacologic strategies can be discerned at present. (At the same time, other pharmacological approaches could also be successful, for instance, the development of drugs that enhance the energy supply to potentially degenerative neurons.)

The first strategy involves general growth factors. Characterized growth factors, or their synthetic analogues, may be used to specifically affect certain cell populations in the brain and spinal cord. There are strong indications that in addition to its peripheral action (114) nerve growth factor (NGF) may also act centrally, and, more specifically, may affect cholinergic neurons in the brain. These neurons, which use the neurotransmitter acetylcholine, seem to require a continuing source of NGF to survive. If for some reason, e.g., as a result of degeneration or injury, the production, or transport, of NGF is interrupted, the nerve cells degenerate approximately within two weeks (87). In general, it may be expected that mimicking the influence of naturally occurring growth factors may provide a lead in the development of effective new drugs to treat both neuro-degenerative diseases and nervous system injury.

Serendipity continues to play an important role in the development of new drugs. In research on factors not directly shown to influence the development or maintenance of the nervous system, it has been observed that cell surface components -including gangliosides affect plasticity. The second strategy involves these cell surface components. Gangliosides, in particular monosialoganglioside (GM1), seem to play a prominent role in the regulation of neuronal growth in the developing and adult nervous system, both during physiological conditions and after cell damage (125). Gangliosides have been associated with increased survival of damaged neurons and most probably also with promotion of lesion-induced sprouting (109). Furthermore, there is evidence that gangliosides and growth factors interact. According to this model, gangliosides enhance the efficacy of growth factors. They may function as a potentiator of trophic factors (124).

Recent developments in a number of research laboratories thus indicate a considerable potential for trophic factors in the treatment of neurodegenerative diseases and nervous system injury. However, the clinical efficacy of trophic factors has, so far, not been proven. Major problems using these drugs in the nervous system involve the route of administration and the bioavailability of the drug at the site of degeneration or lesion. A major problem is devising methods for passage through barriers surrounding neural tissue.

The Blood Brain Barrier (BBB)

The BBB limits passage of many molecules, including drugs, from blood to the extracellular fluids of the brain and vise versa. Its function is to secure a constant internal milieu. This task is important as small fluctuations in concentrations, even of endogenous substances such as hormones, might result in uncontrolled nervous activity. Electron microscopy revealed that the endothelial cells (cells forming the lining of the capilaries)of brain capillaries are joint by 'tight junctions'. The outer layers of two adjoining cells merge to physically join them. As a result a continuous wall is formed, the BBB.

The BBB's characteristics, though essential for life, often are the limiting factor for pharmacological treatment of brain disorders. It is difficult, if not impossible, to get therapeutic concentrations of drugs through the barrier. However, it is known that the barrier is not impenetrable, the brain needs nutrients to survive. Information on transport routes and mechanisms of these nutrients can be of use for design of drugs with improved penetrating characteristics.

Lipid soluble substances can diffuse into the brain, this explains the central effects of such substances as nicotine, ethanol and heroin. Essential nutrients, such as glucose and aminoacids, are less lipid-soluble. Specific transporters, proteins that 'recognize' one substance, act as a pump for these molecules.

As many, essential, drugs have a low lipid solubility, administration to the brain generally entails one of two strategies. Either the BBB is temporarily lowered, or it must be circumvented. Recent tests using sugar solutions to open the barrier are positive and potentially important to enhance efficacy of treatment. The fact that lowering the sugar levels results in an immediate re-closure, trapping the drug inside, may even improve outcome.

Injection into the cerebrospinal fluid is the most direct way to bypass the BBB. A more elegant concept combines the selective permeability of the BBB with the brain's metabolic properties. Some

drugs exist which are able to enter the brain rapidly, and are subsequently modified into active metabolites incapable of recrossing the barrier. For example, this is the case with L-Dopa, which is modified to its active metabolite dopamine, showing sustained effects. While - generally speaking - the properties of the BBB make treatment of brain disorders a difficult task, this concept uses these characteristics to its advantage. In future, development of drugs functioning on the basis of this principle opens up new possibilities for treatment (62).

Parkinson's Disease and Alzheimer's Disease. Research on trophic factors may eventually lead to new pharmacological treatments of neuro-degenerative diseases, such as Parkinson's disease and Alzheimer's disease (87). Within the context of plasticity, various concepts concerning the path of physiology of such degenerative diseases have been put forward. The cells afflicted may show insufficient functioning of their receptors, or the supply of neurotrophic factors may be hampered, either due to a lack of production, an autoimmune deficiency, or as a result of neurotoxic or viral agents. Pharmacological treatments, then, should aim at enhancing the trophic factor/degenerating neuron interaction, either by additional supply of trophic factors or by increasing their efficacy. Since an acceptable animal model does not exist at present, especially not in the case of Alzheimer's disease, research findings will have to be corroborated step-by-step on human material in which the disease has been confirmed by pathological examination (1; 126) .

Early diagnosis seems essential for effective therapy based on growth factor action. With current techniques, diagnosis can only be made after severe cell loss, as no clinical manifestation of the disease is clearly visible until that moment. New imaging and behavioral diagnostic techniques may be able to considerably reduce the period between the onset and the detection of the disease. One of the issues meriting close examination is how to determine the target group for early diagnosis or screening. Ultimately, postmortem neuropathological confirmation of the disease process is necessary.

Central Nervous System Injury. In lesions due to trauma, trophic factors are considered to be important for the regrowth of damaged cells, counteracting secondary cell loss, or enhancing collateral sprouting (51; 32). When central nervous system injury occurs, the circuitry of neuronal connections is interrupted. Soon after the initial trauma, the remaining tissue proceeds to deteriorate, resulting in the progressive death of partially damaged neurons near the lesion. This progressive cell death is probably caused by a detrimental biochemical environment (64).

After trauma, glia cells proliferate and form a barrier around the lesion. This barrier was thought to prevent regeneration. However, it has been observed that these glia cells also help spared neurons deal with the injury, for instance, by the regulation of ionic balances and by building excess amino acids. These glial cells also release trophic factors, but their efficacy is considered to be limited. In addition, it takes some time before the production of trophic factors is started. Thus, the initial balance between neurotrophic and neurotoxic substances (e.g. free fatty acid metabolites and excitatory amino acids) is detrimental. Pharmacological treatments are aimed at inducing high neurotrophic and low neurotoxic levels. Intracerebral injections of growth factors enhance neuronal survival and injections of purified gangliosides reduce behavioral deficits (110). For instance, GM1 appears to be important for post-lesion cell sparing and regeneration in the central nervous system. Daily treatment with GM1, for a two week period, has been shown to reduce post-injury behavioral symptoms. In part, these trophic factors rescue neurons from dying. The effectiveness of treatment is thus partly determined by the duration of the period between damage and the start of treatment. The lag-time should be as short as possible. In addition, for these treatments to be clinically successful, the neurons spared by trauma or saved by selective death must maintain some behavioral function. In the spinal cord, 10 percent of the axons in the ventral funiculus is already sufficient to sustain near normal locomotion (8; 83). Thus, relatively few neurons saved will greatly strengthen the functional regeneration process.

Peripheral Nerve Injury. For years it has been known that repair of damaged nervous tissue is relatively less complicated in the peripheral nervous system. Much research is directed towards biochemically enhancing the regeneration of peripheral nerves. One example is the use of neuropeptides from the ACTH-MSH family. These neuropeptides have been shown to facilitate recovery of sensory and motor function after peripheral injury (39).

Local administration of the peptide at the site of the nerve damage by means of diffusion from a biodegradable polymer tube remarkably enhances neurite outgrowth and subsequent recovery (40). Such a delivery system releases the trophic factors in a continuous way for an extended period, protects and directs the axons, and keeps the naturally produced trophic factors close to the lesion. It creates a 'permissive' milieu that allows faster recovery and bridging over extended distances.

Furthermore, these peptides have been shown to protect the nervous system against neurotoxic side-effects of chemotherapy as used in various cancers. Clinical trials using this peptide have recently been started. The clinical significance could be profound, since treatment with growth promoting substances seems easier to conduct, less costly than transplants, and would avoid possible ethical problems inherent in the use of human tissue for transplantation. Both in neurodegenerative disorders and with injury, results are best when intervention is started as early as possible.

Environmental Interventions

Environmental factors play an important role in establishing and maintaining nervous system plasticity. Nutrition, drugs, alcohol, environmental agents, or occupational exposure to toxic agents may influence nervous system plasticity (24; 54). So far, knowledge concerning the **direct** influence of these environmental factors on plasticity in the adult nervous system is relatively scarce, except for their effects on plastic phenomena such as learning and their stimulation of plastic processes due to neuronal injury. In future, however, environmental factors may be found to directly influence the loss of trophic factors responsible for the maintenance of particular types of neurons (17; 19).

Another type of environmental factor in plasticity concerns stimulation and deprivation. Classical experiments concerning the effects of visual deprivation were described in the previous chapter. Questions regarding the consequences of use and disuse are also of importance in relation to nervous system plasticity. In peripheral target organs, for example, the phenomenon of muscle atrophy due to the destruction of muscle nerves is well-known (122). Furthermore, social deprivation has been shown to influence learning, aggression, or sexual behavior (27). Recent studies in rats have even indicated a potential reduction in life span. Many studies concerning an 'enriched' environment indicate changes in anatomy and biochemistry of the brain, and subsequent behavioral changes.

Although beyond the scope of this report, the importance of physical and social environmental factors in the human developing brain has been studied much more extensively. Particularly during embryonic and fetal stages, the human brain is in its most plastic state, and thus vulnerable to environmental factors. Neurotoxic exposure may result in developmental disorders, which may in part be prevented by environmental interventions (59).

The environmental interventions described in the following sections are interventions in both the physical and social environment with the aim to ameliorate or enhance human health.

Alzheimer's Disease. Research in elderly healthy and demented subjects suggests that some measures of brain functioning may be influenced by environmental factors (121). However, studies on the effects of environmental interventions upon mental well-being of demented subjects are relatively scarce. Environmental interventions may be classified as either physical activation or behavioral programs (92). A well-designed study concerning the effects of activation therapy in demented subjects is being carried out in the Netherlands. Behavioral programs can take a variety of forms. One strategy, reality orientation, is aimed at promoting the re-use of neglected functions or the development of new behavioral strategies in order to compensate for deficits in isolated elderly patients. The exact effects of this program have as yet not been established. It has been argued that this intervention might be of greater value to elderly demented patients which are not yet hospitalized. In one study, patients attending a geriatric psychiatry day hospital did show improvement on tests of orientation and mental impairment following this therapy (63).

Parkinson's Disease. Only a small group of studies have explored how those with Parkinson's disease adapt to their disease (67; 112). Hyman identified personality and interpersonal factors that have deleterious effects on patients' well-being. Patients who had low self-esteem, believed that there were no possibilities for cure, willingly accepted the sick role, avoided social contact, and were infantalized by their families were likely to be depressed and demoralized by the disease. Singer found that patients who accept their disease calmly, have high expectations for themselves, and regard their families as having realistic expectations for them, were more likely to be active, socially engaged, and in good spirits after the initation of L-Dopa treatment. Singer's work gives encouragement to the view that patients' status and response to treatment are influenced by attitudes and personal relationships.

An important reason to expand the range of psychological, social, and behavioral factors in studies of Parkinson's disease is that it addresses the ways in which patients strive to overcome, frequently with success, their disabilities and limitations. There are virtually no data on how the very substantial proportion of Parkinson patients who do not have any psychological disorders live with the disease or how it has affected their lives. The identification of factors associated with effective adaptation may provide clues about the factors implicated in psychological distress and may suggest ways to help patients who have problems (35).

Stern et al. survey clinical observations dealing with the ability of those with Parkinson's disease to develop new behavioral strategies to overcome their motor disabilities with success (118). Studies in cats with dysfunctioning basal ganglia, as an animal model of Parkinson's disease, are also promising in this respect (31). Apparently, the healthy cortex enables the person with Parkinson's disease to use external stimuli and to construct a compensatory activity for effects of the disease.

Of the various environmental factors that might contribute to the cause of Parkinson's disease, attention has largely focused on the possible role of infectious and toxic agents (25). Evidence of viral infection of the central nervous system has been reported in populations of those with Parkinson's disease, but none of these claims has been confirmed. A slow or latent virus could have a causal role. Recently, it has been shown that certain coronaviruses have the potential to elicit chronic central nervous system disease in animals by causing a persistent CNS infection of the substantia nigra, i.e., a key structure in Parkinson's disease (48). The potential of these viruses to cause postencephalic parkinsonism or Parkinson's disease is beginning to be explored.

Exposure to drugs that deplete dopamine or block dopamine receptors leads, in man, to the clinical syndrome of parkinsonism. Though this phenomenon is reversible in most cases, it can have significant relevance in elderly in whom dopamine production falls with advancing age. In the elderly, such drugs can evoke overt parkinsonism or unmask latent idiopathic disease.

An important new toxin which produces a syndrome resembling nearly all of the changes seen in classical Parkinson's disease is 1-methyl-4-phenyl-1,2,5,6-tetrahydropyridine (MPTP). Both chemists who synthesized compounds requiring preparation of MPTP or its derivatives, and addicts who injected themselves intravenously with self-manufactured pethidine analogues including MPTP developed Parkinson's disease (79). The extent to which Parkinson's disease induced by insecticides, fungicides, and herbicides is also due to MPTP and/or its metabolites needs investigation (16). At any rate, there obviously are neurotoxic compounds with extreme potency and selectivity that can cause Parkinson's disease and can affect the plasticity of the nervous system.

Environmental hazards such as MPTP may not be detected for years. The exposure can occur many years before onset of symptoms. This highlights the importance of prevention through environmental regulation.

Chapter IV – Future Health Care Consequences and Social Implications

The areas of research included under neuroplasticity are germane to a large number of health-related problems. Rapid developments in plasticity research may lead to new methods of prevention and treatment of such problems within the coming decades. The previous Chapter discussed the potential future applicability of such developments for Alzheimer's disease, Parkinson's disease, and injury involving nervous system trauma. Obviously, future technological applications will have large implications for health and the quality of life of those afflicted with these problems. In addition, they may influence the organization and delivery of health care to a considerable extent.

Health Care Consequences

Technological change is one of the important factors influencing the health care system. Other major factors that affect health care delivery include changing patterns of health needs and health demands.

Chapter III briefly presented an overview of the incidence and prevalence of the diseases addressed in this case-study. In general, these diseases exert heavy demands on health care resources. For example, the majority of people who sustain nervous system trauma are under 35 years of age. As a result of intensive medical care, their life expectancy has increased; however, a large number of people remain more or less severely disabled (with paralysis, for example). The demand for health care (and for other social services) is therefore often large.

Neurodegenerative diseases, such as Alzheimer's disease and Parkinson's disease, are correlated with advanced age. Consequently, their prevalence can be projected to rise in the future, due to an aging population. At present, a relatively large fraction of these patients are institutionalized. For example, it was found that in one 500 bed geriatric nursing home in New York, 65 percent of the residents met clinical and mental status criteria for dementia (72). Extrapolating from past trends, the need for long term care in the future will increase dramatically.

Straightforward extrapolation is highly unrealistic, however. Social, economic, and technological forces may influence and change the trend towards institutionalization. For example, if application of the results of plasticity research, such as transplantation or new pharmacological agents, could delay institutionalization for 5 years, the consequences for nursing homes in the Netherlands would be considerable. The STG scenario study on aging made illustrative calculations to indicate the possible magnitude of such effects (120). The calculations should not be seen as exact predictions, since the many dynamics of the disease and its care system have not been taken into account. The results indicate that such a delay of institutionalization would decrease the number of demented persons in Dutch nursing homes by 26 percent up to the year 2000, in comparison with a no-change scenario.

Table 4 Number of patients of 65 and older in nursing homes with dementia as principal diagnosis.

	1981, 1982, 1983 (average)	2000 without delay of institutionalization	2000 with delay of institutionalization
Female	9279	14144	10225
Male	2699	3587	2816
Total	11978	17731	13041

Source: STG Report on Aging (120)

Thus, if the institutionalization could be delayed by 5 years, the number of demented persons in nursing homes would increase 9 percent by the year 2000 compared to the 1980's. If it cannot be delayed, the number of demented persons in nursing homes would increase 48 percent by the year 2000. The consequences for the number of nursing homes needed and subsequent health expenditures are apparent.

The analysis made in this project, however, leads to the conclusion that although progress in plasticity research is very rapid, large-size clinical applications for the disease categories analyzed are not to be expected in the near future. It is impossible to predict sudden breakthroughs, but if such breakthroughs do not occur, it seems safe to assume that it will be ten to twenty years before effective treatment or preventive tools will be available for such diseases as Alzheimer's disease. In view of the fact that new large scale applications do not seem to be likely in the near future, an attempt to quantify the consequences of research advances for the organization of the health care system is at present not indicated.

The introduction of new technologies on a more limited scale for the diseases analyzed may be expected in the nearer future. The introduction of these technologies raises a number of specific issues. The introduction of nervous tissue transplants, as an experimental procedure, is associated with questions concerning safety and efficacy, in addition to ethical and legal issues (see below). As in the case of all significant new health care technologies, well-designed clinical studies of efficacy and safety are imperative before widespread applications can be considered. New drugs based on neurotrophic factors will be regulated for safety and efficacy as are any new drugs.

Environmental interventions may affect the organization and delivery of care, as well as having broader social and economic implications. In Parkinson's disease, the identification of psychosocial variables associated with effective adaptation and response to treatment may lead to new opportunities to promote health. Such behavioral and social interventions would require changes in the approach of health care professionals. However careful assessment of their effectiveness is needed. In the case of Alzheimer's disease, the introduction of the concept of an 'enriched environment' needs to be considered. More research is needed, since programs of sensory stimulation have not been shown to defenitive reverse impairment associated with dementia. If, however, such programs are proven to influence health status in addition to quality of life, this may very well lead to changes in the functioning of nursing homes. Today, nursing homes often do not offer a very stimulating environment in terms of architecture, interior design, daily schedules, and personal relationships, due partly to reasons of efficiency. Reforms of long-term care institutions may very well increase costs. Society must decide how much the potential benefits are worth and if it is willing to support cost increases.

Social and Economic Consequences

In the future, plasticity research and its technological applications may have social and economic consequences. New preventive and treatment measures in the area of nervous system trauma could decrease overall costs. Especially in this area, new approaches may also alleviate lost worker productivity and its economic cost (99). The costs of new interventions in the neurodegenerative diseases are uncertain. As mentioned in the previous section, cost-effectiveness analyses of any proposed intervention are desirable.

In philosophical, religious, and ethical sense, the brain, and its relationship to the concept of mind, represents a symbolic value in many cultures. Neurosciences research can also be considered within this broader frame of reference. Future developments in neurosciences research may have fundamental humanistic implications. For example, they could lead to changing concepts relating to the nature of consciousness, freedom of choice, causal determinacy, and the fundamental relation of mind to matter and to brain mechanisms (115). In the last decades, plasticity research has helped change the concept of the human brain from a static to a more dynamic one. The implications of such changes can be far-reaching in the long run.

For example, one area of plasticity research investigates mechanisms of learning at a number of levels of the nervous system. Improved knowledge may contribute to the understanding of certain forms of learning disabilities and may improve methods of teaching children with these disabilities. In a broader sense, new insights concerning learning and memory may lead to better methods of teaching, and change the education system.

Neurotoxic substances (see also Chapters I and III), such as drugs, nutrition, environmental agents, and occupational exposure, can result in nervous system disease and affect plasticity. In the case of Parkinson's disease, for instance, a number of studies have implicated pesticides, insecticides, herbicides, and drugs. Many heavy metals, pesticides, and organic solvents influencing the nervous system and its plasticity have been identified, leading to improved industrial and environmental controls (99). Neurotoxic effects of numerous substances have not yet been discovered, however, partly due to the difficulties in detecting neural damage and the often long period of time between first exposure and identification of the first definite symptoms. As neurotoxic effects of both new and established substances are discovered, new regulations will be needed.

Ethical and Legal Aspects

There are legal and ethical issues that result from developments in plasticity research. A central issue in experimental research and treatment is the doctrine of informed consent; within this case-study, the ability of demented persons to give informed consent needs specific consideration (81). Demented persons in most cases cannot adequately judge the risks involved in research, and thus lack the necessary legal capacity and/or comprehension (80). Ethical and legal issues center around the question who should decide whether these patients should be part of clinical trials, and what the standards should be for ensuring protection of their rights.

If only mentally incompetent people are available, consent of a legal guardian must be obtained (38). Ethics Committees can also be developed to review and consult in the case of decision-making for those who lack the capacity to decide (101).

At present, a law on medical experiments with human subjects is being prepared in the Netherlands. This law will include general rules to protect the interests of those who lack legal decision-making capacity. One part of such a law could set up a national 'Ethics Committee' that could develop specific guidelines on a number of complex ethical issues, such as selection criteria for transplant procedures (107). (In the Netherlands, present ethics committee function primarily on a hospital level.) The issue of research on demented people merits specific consideration by such a Committee.

Guidelines have been developed dealing with the use of fetal tissue in research, implicitly including transplants of fetal nervous tissue (95; 57). The use of fetal tissue in experimental treatment is a complex and controversal issue. Ethical and legal issues center around the questions if fetal tissue may be used, and, if so, under what conditions.

In the coming five years the ethical and legal questions should center around the use of fetal tissue in a limited number of **experimental** procedures. In the long run, however, alternatives to fetal tissue, such as cell culture lines, may be developed. Research on such alternatives is already done and preliminary results are promising. Large scale clinical application of transplants using fetal tissue, thus, never may occur.

An extensive discussion of the various ethical positions can be found in the literature (95; 9; 65). In the Netherlands, the Health Council concluded that fetal tissue from abortions or miscarriages could be used for scientific purposes under certain conditions (57; 53). The Health Council report confines itself to pregnancies terminated before a maximum of 24 weeks. A central premise in the report is that moral considerations apply to all who have human genetic material and that fetal tissue should be treated respectfully and with dignity (95). The guidelines of the Health Council address both conditions for use and supply of fetal tissue. The summary of these guidelines is included in this report as Appendix B.

A key issue in the report concerns criteria of death. The conclusion is that it is permissible to carry out medical research on fetuses which show no signs of life at birth (no brainstem reflexes), and that fetal tissue that shows signs of life may only be used after it has become impossible to activate the brainstem reflexes and specifically the trigeminus reflex.

Another important ethical and legal issue covered in the report is informed consent by the women. The report differentiates the consent procedure in the case of miscarriage and induced abortion. In the case of miscarriage, informed consent is required from the woman, and in appropriate cases, her partner should be informed. In the case of induced abortion, the woman should be informed of the possibility of fetal tissue being used for medical research and given the opportunity to object. This conclusion has been criticized for inconsistency, and is considered not justified ethically (18; 9). There seems no justification for differentiation; informed consent should be required in both cases.

The Health Council report also concludes that an institutional ethics committee should oversee the use of fetal tissue in research.

Chapter V – Summary and Conclusions

Summary

The area of neurosciences research is rapidly evolving. In the past decades considerable progress has been made in understanding nervous system functioning, including the mechanisms involved in neurological, behavioral, and communicative disorders.

In the first chapter of this report some promising directions of research and technology development within the neurosciences have been highlighted; the field shows to have a high scientific and technological potential. For example, research on neuropeptides may lead to new effective drugs for the treatment of a variety of mental and nervous system diseases. In general, while there has been a considerable increase in knowledge, one can argue that the field is still early in its development. The major clinical applications of many of these research findings lie years ahead in the future. In the long run, research in the neurosciences promises to provide tools for the prevention, diagnosis, and effective treatment of nervous system disorders.

The neurological, communicative, and behavioral disorders afflict a significant part of the present-day population in industrialized countries. Due to the aging of the population these disorders can be expected to increase in prevalence in the coming decades. The clinical significance of new technological applications from neurosciences research is thus potentially profound. In addition to the potential impact on health status, such new technologies also promise to greatly affect the nature of the health care system, the costs of the system, and even the broader society.

As neurosciences is such a vast field, in this project one specific area - the **plasticity** of nervous tissue was selected for in-depth assessment. Plasticity refers to the properties of the nervous system by which it regenerates, repairs, or reorganizes itself. The nervous system is now seen to have a very dynamic nature. It can change in response to altered conditions inside or outside the organism. The ability of the nervous system to change its activity as a result of previous experience or in response to disease and injury is called neural plasticity.

The focus in this case study is on the **probabilities** of improvements in prevention and treatment of certain nervous system disorders (Alzheimer's disease, Parkinson's disease and injury involving nervous system trauma), resulting from plasticity research. The potential technological applications of plasticity research include transplantation, pharmaceutical developments, and environmental interventions.

During the last few years **nervous tissue transplantation** has been carried out with increasing frequency, especially in rodents (rats), and has attracted considerable interest in the medical profession and the public. Nervous tissue transplantation is a valuable research tool, and the success of recent experiments has suggested that it might also be clinically useful. Applications have been proposed both for the neurodegenerative diseases and for nervous tissue injury through trauma.

The **primary** importance of neuronal transplants currently is in their use as a research tool. This is particularly true since the cause of most neurodegenerative diseases is unknown. Transplants of nerve tissue thus produce valuable knowledge about the functioning of the nervous system, which eventually may contribute to the development of definitive preventive and treatment methods.

As to the **potential clinical applications** of transplants in neurodegenerative diseases, one of the major questions is if transplants will affect the underlying disease process. Within the area of neurodegenerative diseases, the distinction needs to be made between localized and more general brain diseases. Neural transplants may have a clinical role in treating certain localized brain diseases. For example, in the case of Parkinson's disease, which results from loss of certain types of nerve cells, the first experimental grafts in humans have already been done. In the coming years many studies on the safety and the effectiveness in nonhuman primates will be needed to determine the exact clinical applicability of neural transplants. The potential therapeutic use of transplants in general brain diseases, such as Alzheimer's disease, seems to be limited. The possibility of transplantation in the more general brain diseases must await deeper analysis of the disease process. Treating all symptoms of a complex disease with a single type of graft, however, seems to be improbable (50). In addition to these technical limitations, the future prevalence of Alzheimer's disease makes large-scale clinical utilization of transplantation less likely.

The clinical significance of transplants will probably be greater with nervous system injury, both peripheral and central. One of the important reasons for this conclusion is that the cause of the lesion is often the result of trauma and no underlying disease process is involved. Applications of transplants in the peripheral nervous system seem promising. Good clinical functional results have been obtained using autologous nerve grafting techniques. In addition to nerve tissue, various kinds of artificial substances - such as polymers have been used to 'bridge' gaps and stimulate regeneration of nerve fibers. With regard to spinal cord injuries, various transplantation strategies may be used in the future to restore function below the lesion. Research on 'locomotion-generators' and efforts towards constructing an unbroken pathway from the site of the injury to the target muscle may lead to practical clinical applicability. Intracerebral transplants might in future offer promise in the case of certain focal injuries. Much more research is needed, however, before clinical application can be considered.

Research on nervous system plasticity will most likely result in a number of **new pharmacological agents**. Several types of natural substances that regulate growth and cell survival have been identified, including various growth factors and different cell surface components. The first trophic factor to be identified was Nerve Growth Factor (NGF), for this discovery the 1986 Nobel Prize in Physiology or Medicine was awarded to Levi-Montalcini. In the last decade, many more trophic factors have been identified. On the basis of this knowledge, two major pharmacological strategies can be discerned.

- Characterized growth factors, or their synthetic analogues, may be used to specifically affect certain cell populations in the brain and spinal cord.
- Cell surface components, including gangliosides, also have been observed to affect plasticity. Gangliosides, for instance, seem to play a prominent role in the regulation of neuronal growth in the developing and adult nervous system, both under normal physiological conditions and after cell damage. Recent developments in a number of research laboratories indicate a vast potential for growth factors and cell surface components in the treatment of both neurodegenerative diseases and injury. Pharmacological treatment of Parkinson's disease and Alzheimer's disease could aim at enhancing the interaction between the trophic factor and degenerating neuronal tissue, either by giving an additional supply of trophic factors or by increasing their efficacy. Pharmacological treatment after lesions due to trauma is directed towards inducing high neurotrophic levels. Injection of growth factors seems to enhance neuronal survival and injection of gangliosides seems to reduce behavioral deficits.

Early diagnosis is essential for effective therapy based on trophic factor action. Both in neurodegenerative diseases and in injury, results are best when intervention is started as early as possible. With nervous system trauma, early treatment may prevent secondary cell loss, which probably is due to a hostile biochemical environment. New brain imaging and behavioral diagnostic techniques are important with regard to the neurodegenerative diseases as they may considerably reduce the period between the onset and the detection of disease.

The clinical significance of pharmacological treatment could be profound as treatment with trophic substances seems easier to conduct, less costly than transplants, and would avoid possible ethical problems inherent in the use of human tissue for transplantation.

Environmental factors play an important role in establishing and maintaining nervous system plasticity. Thus, interventions in both the physical and social environment may be used to ameliorate or enhance human health.

Both intrinsic and external factors such as motor and sensory experience, or social interactions establish and maintain plasticity. The importance of external factors has especially been shown by stimulation and deprivation experiments in animals. For example, animal studies concerning an 'enriched' environment indicate changes in anatomy and biochemistry of the brain, and subsequent behavioral changes. Research on elderly healthy and demented subjects suggests that brain and behavioral functioning can indeed be influenced by interactions with the general environment. For example, socially stimulating environments allow more normal functioning, even in brain-damaged people. In addition, nutritional factors, drugs, alcoholics, environmental agents, or occupational exposure to toxic agents may influence nervous system plasticity. In future, it may be possible that environmental factors will be found to directly influence the loss of trophic factors, which are responsible for the maintenance of particular types of neurons, and thereby influence the pathogenesis of degenerative diseases. Increased research into possible links between environmental factors and loss of neuroplasticity is needed. Scientific findings in this area may lead to new regulation of chemicals, drugs, and other potentially toxic agents.

Generally speaking, environmental interventions have few, if any, side effects. Their potential in promoting normal functioning of people with nervous system disorders has not been given adequate attention, however. While more research is needed, it seems clear that the potential of environmental and social interventions in this area is considerable.

Although progress in plasticity research is very rapid, large-scale clinical applications for the disease categories discussed in this report cannot be expected within the coming decade. However, when new clinical applications emerge, their implications for health and the delivery of health care will be considerable. For instance, if the application of results of plasticity research could delay the institutionalization because of dementia for five years, rough calculations indicate that the number of demented persons in Dutch nursing homes would decrease by 26 percent in the year 2000, compared with a no-change scenario (120).

Chapter IV of this report also highlighted a number of social and ethical consequences of plasticity research. In the area of transplantation, for instance, the ethical implications of using embryonic or fetal tissue have been discussed.

Conclusions

Progress in neurosciences research is rapid and promises to remain so in the future. Future technological applications of neurosciences research can be expected to have large implications for health, the delivery of health care, and the broader social system. This case study focuses on plasticity research regarding a number of disease categories, and these conclusions relate specifically to this area of research. They may, however, be of broader relevance to the general field of neurosciences.

These considerations indicate the importance of monitoring developments in plasticity research. While the exact timing of advances cannot be predicted, they seem almost certain to come and their consequences may be considerable. For this reason, iterative examination of developments in this field and their potential consequences will be needed. In five years a follow-up of this prospective assessment, involving a more 'quantitative analysis' seems to be indicated.

As technological applications of plasticity research appear, they need to be carefully evaluated. Transplants of nervous tissue already being done illustrate the necessity and challenge of careful evaluation. Environmental interventions gaining visibility also need careful evaluation before they become the accepted standard for clinical care.

Plasticity research also raises a number of ethical and legal issues. In particular, the issue of informed consent by demented persons needs to be considered. In Chapter IV, standards are given for protection of the rights of demented persons.

Transplantation of fetal and embryonic tissue also raises special ethical and legal questions. Standards for this area have already been developed in a report from the Health Council (57). These standards seem adequate except for modifications suggested in this report dealing with informed consent from the mother.

The stage of development of the field of neurosciences is such that new and important findings are appearing at a rapid rate. At the same time, the field could be more effective and productive if certain changes were made. By its nature, neurosciences research is interdisciplinary. In the coming years, it will be necessary to foster and increase interdisciplinary research, including fundamental research, clinical research, and epidemiological research. Certain types of specialized expertise will need to be strengthened for optimal functioning of the field (for example, neuropathology, biological psychiatry, and experimental neurology).

In the previous chapters, the importance of early diagnosis for future therapeutic progress has been stressed. This underscores the need for adequate access to specialized technological resources, including medical imaging devices, immunological techniques, and behavioral techniques. Human experimental research concerning the brain and behavior should be especially stimulated. The disorders addressed in this report manifest themselves in the form of behavioral changes and dysfunctioning. Diagnosis depends on an accurate analysis of such behavioral changes, e.g. deficits of attention, motor- and planning functions, perceptual functions, language processes, and memory processes. The effects of interactions with regard to plasticity likewise need to be measured by neuropsychological techniques. The development of more refined instruments for the measurement of these psychological functions seems promising in this respect. Furthermore, a development that could be of particular utility for all research groups active in the field of neurosciences, would be a general brain bank, since there is no acceptable animal experimental model for a number of brain diseases. Each research step needs to be checked on human brain material. The Alzheimer Brain Bank in Amsterdam is a good start for such a development. Quite a number of requests have already been received to extend the Bank with material from patients with such diseases as schizophrenia, mental retardation, Parkinson's disease, multiple sclerosis, and Down's syndrome.

Appendixes

APPENDIX A TECHNICAL ASPECTS OF NERVOUS TISSUE TRANSPLANTATION

Developmental biologists have long employed transplantation techniques to study normal processes in development and regeneration. Such techniques have been applied mainly in non-mammalian vertebrates and invertebrate animals. Compared with other transplantation procedures in vertebrates, neural transplantation has proven to be a more difficult and more limited procedure. However, in the long run, neural transplants might be even more successful. Although much remains to be solved, neural transplants suffer less from host rejection than other grafts, probably because of the immunologically unique nature of the brain. The brain lacks lymphatic vessels and lymph nodes (which play a critical function in the immune response) and is surrounded by the 'blood-brain barrier,' which decreases the access of the immune system to foreign tissue in the brain. The relative lack of rejection, however, could also be a result of unique characteristics of nerve cells. Most cells carry large molecules with antigenic properties on their surface. The antigens on cells from other animals or people are identified by the immune system of the recipient as 'foreign'. These antigens are rare or absent on most neurons (45).

In a majority of studies dealing with neural transplantation, fetal brain tissue is used as donor material. Neonatal grafts survive less well, whereas adult mammalian CNS neurons do not survive at all. With respect to fetal brain grafts, transplants have been reported to survive in nearly every brain region. An important consideration is the stage of development of the donor tissue, allowing a relatively short critical period during which optimal transplantation of a given region can be performed.

Gage and Bjorklund note that two principal techniques have been used to graft fetal CNS tissue to previously denervated striatal or hippocampal regions (11):

1. the 'solid graft technique' involves the transplantation of solid pieces of tissue to a surgically prepared transplantation cavity in which the graft is placed in direct contact with the denervated striatum or hippocampus. The environment of the graft is enriched in this technique.
2. the 'cell suspension technique' involves injection of dissociated cell suspensions into the depth of the brain. Small amounts of the suspension can be stereotactically injected, allowing precise and multiple placements of the cells.

One important issue in neural transplantation is the specificity of the transplant. In other words, are transplants limited to innervating their normal projection sites or can they innervate any region of the brain into which they are transplanted? Although some studies suggest that abundant innervation may take place after grafting donor tissue into regions other than its own origin, following grafting there is an ordered specificity in the pattern of reinnervation. In addition to CNS transplants, PNS grafting is also being carried out, as well as transplantation of the adrenal medulla, containing chromaffin cells. These latter cells are of interest as they originate from the neural crest, but in the adrenal medulla function as endocrine cells releasing catecholamines. However, after grafting into the brain or the eye chamber, chromaffin cells lose their glandular appearance and start to form processes, finally resulting in large catecholaminergic neurons.

In addition to studies on survival, morphological appearance and reinnervation progress, the functional competence of grafted neurons is a critical issue. Work done on the functional activity of neuroendocrine transplants, especially grafts taken from the hypothalamus-hypophyseal system, have been done in rodents that have a genetic defect in producing certain neuro-hormones. Grafting of the brain region has led to successful restoration of the endocrine balance in the recipient animal.

More recently, several groups are involved in testing whether neural grafts are capable of influencing cognitive functions of the host animal. In such studies, special attention is focused on the septo-hippocampal complex and the medial frontal cortex. Fetal septal grafts placed near the denervated hippocampus provide a nearly normal cholinergic reinnervation of the hippocampus.

The hippocampus has a special role in learning and memory, and lesions in this area in rats are known to result in severe impairments of both working and spatial memory (45). Furthermore, in a number of recipients such grafts ameliorate the memory disorders normally displayed by rats bearing lesions in the septo-hippocampal pathway.

Of special interest are the studies on the survival and functional activity of grafts placed into the aged brain. Evidence is accumulating to suggest that neural transplants which replace populations of neurons that are diminished or lost during aging are effective in partially reversing the functional and cognitive disorders that accompany the age-related cell loss. Thus, in general, survival of fetal grafts seems in the aged brain as effective as in the young recipient brain.

Why only fetal grafts are successfully transplanted is unsolved. It may be that adult neurons with cell surface markers expressed are rejected more readily. Another possibility is that fetal cells are more resistant to the anoxia produced by the surgical procedure. It remains to be shown what precise mechanism is underlying survival of the graft in the host brain. It is certain that local trophic factors from the host brain are often vital in this respect.

The most intensively studied clinical model of brain tissue transplantation concerns the capability of dopaminergic transplants to ameliorate the motor and sensory deficits resulting from lesions in the nigro-striatal system. Damage to dopaminergic neurons results in a variety of behavioral and motor dysfunctions in animals and humans in the form of Parkinson's disease. The data suggest that fetal substantia nigra grafts innervate the host striatum and spontaneously release sufficient dopamine to reduce dopamine receptor sensitivity and to correct motor abnormalities, displayed by rats bearing lesions in the nigro-striatal pathway.

Recently, biomedical scientists have reversed the symptoms of Parkinson's disease in monkeys by successfully transplanting brain cells (105). Since animal experiments have shown that transplantation of embryonic nervous tissue results in the growth of new neurons, and may even restore dysfunctions inherent in the absence of the latter neurons, this technique may be promising in clinical application to Parkinson's disease.

During brain development glial cells provide a matrix for the growth of neurites. Glia cells in the peripheral nervous system, called Schwann cells, stimulate fibers to grow. During aging, but especially due to injury, the supporting cell matrix may be damaged. CNS regeneration may be limited by lack of an appropriate environment. In several studies peripheral nerve grafts and peripheral glia have been used to stimulate CNS axonal regeneration (45).

With regard to **spinal cord** transplantation the ultimate goal is to find a way of restoring function below the lesion. One approach is to improve the milieu to permit regeneration of the endogenous fibers by transplanting bridge grafts. Another is to provide new cells with an increased capacity to generate neuronal processes. There have also been many attempts to find artificial substances to support the regeneration of nerve fibers. Freed et al. review studies, in which peripheral nerves regenerate through silicone tubes for distances of 10mm (51). Various polymers have been used to bridge gaps in transsected nerves and spinal cord, up to now with varying, but limited success.

In general, the use of transplants as a tool in the therapy for brain trauma or degenerative diseases is based upon the presumption that newly formed connections between graft and host tissue mediate beneficial effects on brain function and behavior. However, such a presumption still awaits experimental documentation. Within the field of neuronal plasticity, transplants are important and new fundamental tools for improving knowledge of the development and repair of neuronal circuitry. Even though the potential clinical use of the technique itself may be further in the future, research on reinnervation and restoration of functional deficits should be strongly encouraged. Such studies should include both the central as well as the peripheral nervous system and should concentrate on properties of the graft itself as well as the host conditions which enable the survival, regrowth and repair of damaged neuronal tissue, including the search for neurotrophic and immunologic factors governing proper acceptance of the graft and proper growth of the axons.

APPENDIX B SUMMARY OF THE DUTCH HEALTH COUNCIL REPORT (1984) CONCERNING THE USE OF FETAL TISSUE FROM ABORTION OR MISCARRIAGES FOR SCIENTIFIC PURPOSES

Summary

The present report examines the question by the State Secretary for Health and Environmental Protection as to whether it is permissible for foetal tissue originating from abortions or miscarriages to be made available for scientific use. If the question was answered in the affirmative, the committee was also to consider whether it was necessary or desirable to establish regulations on the subject.

The report begins with definitions of terminology (chapter 3).

Chapter 4 contains general remarks on the state of science, looking first at the medical and biological background to the use of foetal tissue in various forms of research and treatment. The research areas and the purposes for which foetal tissue and material are used are reviewed, and the arguments for establishing regulations on the use and provision of foetal tissue in particular are considered. The delimitation of the terms of reference is explained: the committee limits itself to making recommendations on the use and supply of tissue and material resulting from a pregnancy terminated spontaneously or artificially up to 24 weeks after conception.

Chapter 5 states the committee's reasons for its views on the criteria for permissible use of foetuses, foetal tissue and foetal material (within the stated time limit). Medical, ethical and legal aspects are considered. This leads to the formulation in chapter 6 of the conditions to which use and supply must be subject and how an ethics committee should apply them. When considering plans for research, it should consider both use and supply in the light of the following conditions.

Conditions for Use

These relate firstly to the protection of tissues and materials resulting from pregnancy, and notably of the foetus, and secondly to the protection of pregnant women, researchers, doctors and members of the nursing and technical staff.

I Protection of tissues and materials resulting from pregnancy, and notably of the foetus

1. Foetal tissue which shows signs of life may only be used for medical research puroposes after it has become impossible to activate the brainstem reflexes and notably the trigeminus reflex. Up to this point, only such action may be undertaken as would be permissible in the case of a viable newly born baby. (Although the commitee confined itself to reporting on pregnancies terminated after a maximum of 24 weeks, it recommends that non-viable foetuses which show signs of life and which originate from pregnancies terminated at a later stage should be treated in the same way for the purposes of this paragraph).

2. It is permissible to carry out medical research on foetuses which show no signs of life upon birth (other than activity in certain organs and cells not externally perceptible).

3. It is permissible to carry out medical research on foetal material (i.e. material resulting from pregnancy other than the foetus itself).

4. It is not permissible to carry out medical research on foetuses which may be capable of functioning as a self-sustaining whole, with the exception of measures which would be permissible in the case of a viable newly born baby.

5. If there is any doubt in ascertaining brain death, advice should be sought from a medical expert not directly involved either in the abortion or in the research.

II Protection of pregnant women, researchers, doctors and nursing and technical staff

1. A doctor at a clinic who is involved in the decision that abortion is indicated should not be the same as the researcher.

2. Doctors, researchers and nursing and technical staff must be informed in advance of the nature of research carried out on foetal tissue.

3. In all questions which face researchers on foetal tissue, including any not referred to in this report, the same general rule should be followed on which this report is based, namely that the foetus should be treated with respect and dignity.

4. No abortion technique may be selected for purposes of medical research which conflicts with the interests of the women concerned. Thus, the interests of the pregnant woman prevail over the aims of the research.

Conditions for Supply

1. Foetal tissue may only be supplied to establishments which have an ethics committee (if necesarry, one appointed for a region). This condition does not apply for diagnostic case studies, e.g. by the pathologist.

2. The rules of conduct which currently apply to corpses at pathology laboratories and obstetrical and gynaecological clinics also apply where tissues and materials originating in pregnancy are supplied.

3. Before the hospital or clinic where the abortion or miscarriage takes place, supplies any foetal tissue to the establishment carrying out the medical research, they should jointly draw up written rules concerning ethical criteria, the purpose of the research, and how foetal tissue is to be obtained and transported.

4. In the case of unwished pregnancy, foetal tissue may be supplied after abortion if and after the woman has been informed of the possibility of foetal tissue being used for medical research, under such conditions that she has the opportunity to object. In the case of a miscarriage or interruption of an initially wished for pregnancy by abortion, tissue may be supplied with the woman's consent; in appropriate cases her husband or partner should be informed, but if he and the woman are unable to agree, the woman should decide. As regards minors, where any decision needs to be taken, this should be done in accordance with the general procedures which are customary for abortions on minors.

5. Doctors and nursing or technical staff should be informed in advance that it is intended that foetal tissue should be supplied to researchers and informed of the nature of the research.

6. Foetal tissue or material should not be supplied for motives of financial gain on the part of a parent, the doctor carrying out the abortion or the researcher; nor should research establishments encourage people to supply such tissue or material with the aid of financial motives.

The committee recommends against incorporating any of these conditions in statutory instruments to which legal sanctions would be attached. However, it considers it desirable that the Inspector of Public Health should monitor future developments in practice in order to be able to take action if they take an undesirable turn.

Obviously, this summary cannot by any means convey all the details dealt with in the individual chapters. It gives only an indication of the issues involved.

APPENDIX C METHOD OF THE STUDY

The need for examining future health care technology was recognized by the Dutch Steering Committee on Future Health Scenarios (STG) in 1984. (The STG is an independent advisory group to the Dutch government set up in 1983 to carry out scenario studies as an aid to long-term health planning). The STG initiated the Project on Future Health Care Technology. The World Health Organization, European Office (EURO), agreed to support the project financially and logistically.

The project had two specific objectives:

1. **To identify future technological developments in health care, with brief descriptions of potential technologies**; and
2. **To carry out prospective assessments of four high priority technologies or areas of technological development.**

The project began in April 1985. A Commission on Future Health Care Technology, made up of 10 members and 5 official observers, was appointed to guide the project. Surveys of experts were carried out in the United States and Europe. The information from the surveys, supplemented by material from the scientific literature and from interviews, was the basis for the overall descriptions of health care technology. The assistance of these many individuals and groups is specifically acknowledged in appendixes to Volumes I and II of this report.

A detailed description of methods for the entire project is presented in an appendix to Volume I of the report. An updated version may be found in Volume II. And each case study contains a methods description specific to that case.

The project plan called for four technologies to be prospectively assessed. In September 1985, the Commission met and endorsed four cases:

1. implications of neurosciences;
2. biotechnology probably examining both monoclonal antibodies and vaccines;
3. laser applications, especially in surgery and in the treatment of vascular disease, especially coronary artery disease; and

4. genetic screening and diagnosis.
Later, with funding from the Ministry of Economic Affairs, medical imaging and home care technology were also developed as case studies.

A working group meeting was held in September 1985 to discuss general considerations in the field of neurosciences. Subsequently, a draft report on Developments in the Regeneration, Repair and Reorganization of Nervous Tissue was written with the assistance of a number of people. Contributions by experts in the field formed the basis of the first chapter. The contributors and members of the working group are acknowledged in the opening pages of this report. The second chapter was drafted by Prof.dr. W.H. Gispen and Prof.dr. F.M. Lopes da Silva.

The implications of plasticity research for health and health-care were discussed in June 1986 by the working group on medical implications of neurosciences. It was decided to concentrate on the possible implications of nervous transplants, pharmacological developments, and environmental intervention for Alzheimer's disease, Parkinson's disease and injury involving nervous tissue trauma.

In a meeting of 24 September 1986, the Commission discussed the draft report on neurosciences. Suggestions for conclusions on the neurosciences case were incorporated into the report together with other changes suggested by reviewers. The conclusions of the neurosciences report were discussed with Prof.dr. D. de Wied and Prof.dr. W.H. Gispen on 19 November 1986. The report was then finalized, sent to reviewers for comments, and revised. The Commission approved the neurosciences report at its meeting of 4 February 1987. After final revisions, the report was submitted to the STG in mid-March 1987.

APPENDIX D GLOSSARY OF TERMS

Acetylcholine: A reversible acetic acid ester of choline, present in the body and having important physiological functions, such as playing a role in the transmission of an impulse/signal of a nerve fiber across a synaptic function.

Acute: In medical care, used to describe a condition that has a sudden onset, sharp rise, and short course (compare **chronic**). In occupational and environmental health, used to describe a disease or injury that is manifest soon after exposure to a hazard.

Affective disorders: Psychological disorders whose symptoms involve a marked change in the patient's mood or emotional state (e.g., manic depression).

Alzheimer disease: A type of dementia most commonly found in elderly persons that is characterized by loss of short-term memory and impairment of the ability to concentrate, think clearly, and speak.

Ambulatory care: Medical services provided to patients who are not hospitalized.

Amino acid: The basic building block of all peptides and proteins.

Amyotrophic lateral sclerosis (ALS): A degenerative disease of the spinal motor neurons controlling skeletal muscles. This disorder most frequently attacks men in their forties, gradually paralyzing them as their motor neurons become increasingly unable to conduct impulses necessary for muscular movement. ALS is fatal, and its cause is unknown. Also known as Lou Gehrig's Disease.

Angiography: Visualization of any blood vessel using X-radiographs after the injection of radiopaque (impervious to the rays) material into the bloodstream.

Artheriography indicates the same technique as angiography when applied to arteries exclusively.

Arteriosclerosis: A condition in which the arterial walls become thickened and hardened. The causes are multiple and complex, and often incompletely known. Also called "hardening of the arteries". See **atherosclerosis**.

Atherosclerosis: A very common form of arteriosclerosis in which deposits of fibrous and cellular tissue, cholesterol, and fat accumulate in large and medium-sized arteries, impeding blood flow.

Autonomic nervous system: That part of the nervous system which is not under voluntary control and which regulates the activity of cardiac muscle, smooth muscle (e.g., in the digestive tract), respiration, glands, a.o..

Axon: The cytoplasmic, slender, cylindrical process of a nerve cell by which impulses are transmitted away from the nerve cell body towards synapses with adjacent cells, where the signal may be passed on. Axons may extend for long distances.

Bioassay: Determination of the active power of a chemical or physical agent by noting its effect on a live animal or an isolated organ preparation. Also called "biological assay".

Biochemical: Refering to biochemistry, the chemistry of living organisms and of vital processes.

Biologics: Medicinal preparations made from living organisms and their products, including serums, vaccines, antigens, antitoxins, etc.

Biopsy: The removal and examination, usually microscopic, of tissue from the living body, in order to establish a precise diagnosis.

Biotechnology: Techniques that use living organisms or substances from organisms to make or modify a product. "New" biotechnology refers to recombinant DNA techniques and other sophisticated devices relying on the ability to harness and manipulate genetic material.

Brain stem: Brain structures collectively forming a stem or stalk between the spinal cord and the base of the brain. It includes the midbrain, pons, and medulla. The brain stem controls many muscular and is also involved in auditory and visual reflexes. The brain stem contains centers controlling such autonomic functions as respiration, blood pressure, gastrointestinal function, arousal, wakefulness and sleep.

Calcium channel blockers: Drugs that block calcium channels in nerve cells and muscle cells, reducing transmitter release in nerve cells and inhibiting contraction in muscle cells. These drugs are used to treat various cardiovascular diseases including angina pectoris, heart attack, arrhythmia, and hypertension.

Carotid bifurcation: The division into two branches of the principal artery in the neck.

Catalysis: Acceleration of a chemical reaction or process produced by the presence of a substance that is not consumed in the course of this reaction or process.

Catalytic: Causing catalysis.

Catecholamine: Group of neuro-transmitters, including dopamine, norepinephrine, and epinephrine.

Cell: The smallest membrane-bound protoplasmic unit consisting of a nucleus and its surrounding cytoplasm, and capable of independent reproduction.

Cell culture: Growth in the laboratory of cells isolated from multicellular organisms. Each cell culture usually consists of one cell type only.

Cell line: Living cells obtained from humans and other animals and cultured under special conditions so that they can multiply indefinitely in vitro.

Cerebral cortex: The convoluted outer layer of the brain which is involved in all higher cognitive, perceptual, and motor functions.

Cerebral infarction: An area of dead tissue in the cerebrum caused by an interruption of blood circulation due to functional constriction or actual obstruction of a blood vessel, hemorrhage, etc. See also **Cerebrum**.

Cerebrovascular disease: A group of diseases affecting or pertaining to the blood vessels of the cerebrum or brain.

Cerebrum: The main portion of the brain, occupying the upper part of the cranial cavity.

Cholesterol: A steroid alcohol present in animal cells and body fluids, important in physiological processes and implicated as a factor in atherosclerosis.

Cholinergic drugs: Drugs that are activated by choline and associated with the synaptic transmission of nerve impulses; such drugs promote bladder contraction.

Chromosome: A structure in the nucleus of animal cells containing DNA.

Chronic: Lingering, lasting, as opposed to acute. A term used to describe persistent disease. Also, in occupational and environmental health, used to describe a disease or injury that is manifest long after exposure to a hazard.

Clone: A group of genetically identical cells or organisms produced asexually from a common ancestor.

Computed tomography (CT) scanner: A diagnostic device combining the X-ray technology with a computer and a cathode ray tube (television-like device) to produce images of cross-sections of the body. Also called "computerized axial tomography (CAT) scanner".

Congenital: Existing at birth.

Congenital abnormality: Any abnormality, whether genetic or not, that is present at birth.

Control group: In a randomized clinical trial this is the group which receives standard treatment, a placebo, or no treatment and with which the group receiving experimental treatment is compared. See **experimental group**.

Cost-benefit analysis (CBA): An analytical technique that compares the costs of a project or a technological application to the resultant benefits, with both costs and benefits expressed by the same measure. This measure is nearly always monetary.

Cost-effectiveness analysis (CEA): An analytical technique that compares the costs of a project or of alternative projects to the resultant benefits, with costs and benefits/effectiveness expressed by different measures. Costs are usually expressed in dollars, but benefits/effectiveness are ordinarily expressed in terms such as "lives saved", "disability avoided", "quality-adjusted life years saved", or any other relevant objective. When benefits or effectiveness are difficult to express in a common metric, they should be (but usually aren't) presented as an "array".

Cost-effectiveness analysis/cost-benefit analysis (CEA/CBA): A composite term used by the U.S. Office of Technology Assessment (OTA) to refer to a family of analytical techniques that are employed to compare costs, effectiveness and benefits of programs or technologies.

CT scanner: See computed tomography (CT) scanner.

Cytopathic: Pertaining to or characterized by abnormal changes in cells.

Dementia: Organic loss of mental function, which may include deterioration of intellectual function, memory loss, and personality changes. Many types of dementia are thought to involve structural and biochemical abnormalities in the nervous system. Alzheimer's disease is one form of dementia.

Depression: A psychiatric syndrome involving dejected moods and often poor sleep and loss of weight. Depression may have genetic and biochemical components. Antidepressant drugs seem to act by affecting neurotransmitters in the brain.

Digital subtraction angiography (DSA): A radiologic tool used for the diagnosis of conditions pertaining to the internal structure of blood vessels. The procedure involves injecting a contrast medium into the patient's veins and then monitoring the medium as it passes through the veins. A computer "subtracts" the images made of the vessels before the injection from the images after the injection in order to give the image of the actual arterial condition.

Disability: A term used to denote the presence of one or more functional limitations. A person with a disability has a limited ability or an inability to perform one or more basic life functions (e.g., walking) at a level considered "typical". Compare to **handicap** and **impairment**.

Disease prevention: Averting the occurence of disease, traditionally characterized as primary, secondary, and tertiary prevention. Primary prevention aims at avoiding disease altogether. Secondary prevention strategies try to detect disease in its early stages of development, with the hope of minimizing deteriation. Tertiary prevention attempts to arrest further deterioration in individuals who already suffer from a disease.

DNA: Deoxyribonucleic acid. The nucleic acid in chromosomes which codes for the genetic information. The molecule is double-stranded helix with two external "backbones" formed by chains of alternating phosphate and sugar (deoxyribose) units and an internal ladder-like structure formed by nucleotide base-pairs held together by hydrogen bonds. The nucleotide base pairs consist of the bases adenine (A), cytosine (C), guanine (G) and thymine (T) whose structures are such that A can hydrogen bond only with T, and C only with G. The sequence of each individual chain can be deduced from knowing that of its partner. This complementarity is the key to the information transmitting capabilities of DNA. (See also **nucleotide** and **gene**.)

Drug: Any chemical or biological substance that may be applied to, ingested by, or injected into humans in order to prevent, treat, or diagnose disease or other medical conditions.

Effectiveness: Same as efficacy (see below) except that it refers to "...average or actual conditions of use".

Efficacy: The probability of benefit to individuals in a defined population from a medical technology applied for a given medical problem under ideal conditions of use.

Electrophoresis: A technique for separating different molecules based on their differential movement in an electric field. The differential movement is a complex function of molecule size, shape, and net electrical charge.

Encephalins: One of the subtypes of endorphins. To date, only two of these substances have been isolated, each composed of five amino acids and differing only in one part of the molecule. When injected into rats, encephalins have a relatively mild painkilling effect and seem to produce strong dependence.

Endorphins: A group of endogenous brain substances (polypeptides) that bind to specific opiate receptors in cells scattered throughout the brain to produce painkilling and euphoric effects similar to those of opium poppy derivatives like morphine and heroin. Endorphins can produce the tolerance and addiction characteristic of opiates. They occur in various forms, including alpha-, beta-, and gamma endorphins and the encephalins. The term derives from "endogenous morphine-like substances".

Enzyme: Any of a group of catalytic proteins that are produced by living cells and that mediate and promote the chemical processes of life without themselves being altered or destroyed.

Epidemiology: The scientific study of the distribution and occurrence of human diseases and health conditions, and of their determinants.

Epidemiologic studies: Studies concerned with the relationships of various factors determining the frequency and distribution of specific diseases in a human community.

Etiologic: Causative.

Etiology: Cause or origin.

Euphoria: The sense of well-being; absense of pain or distress. In psychiatry , an exaggerated sense of well-being.

Experimental group: In a randomized clinical trial, the group receiving the treatment being evaluated for safety and efficacy. The experimental treatment may be a new technology, an existing technology applied to a new problem, or an accepted treatment about whose safety or efficacy there is doubt. Compare **control group**.

Gene: The biologic unit of heredity, self-reproducing and located at a definite position (locus) on a particular chromosome. This basic fundamental unit of heridity is formed by a specific sequence of nucleotide bases in the DNA molecule.

Handicap: Inability to perform one or more life functions (e.g., eating, conversing, working) at a "typical" level, caused by the interaction of an individual's disability with the physical and social environments in which that person is functioning or expected to function. Compare to **disability** and **impairment**.

Hemorrhage: The escape of blood from the blood vessels, either into surrounding tissues or into the environment.

Hippocampus: A curved structure in the limbic system at the core of the brain that is important for learning and the conversion of short- to long-term memory.

Hormone: A chemical substance released into the circulatory system by a gland that has a specific regulatory effect on another organ; functions regulated include metabolism, growth, and the development of secondary sex characteristics (such as breasts, facial hair).

Huntington disease: A rare genetic disease characterized by chronic progressive disorders of movement and mental deterioration culminating in dementia. The disease is transmitted as an autosomal dominant trait, but usually does not manifest itself until a person is between the ages of 30 and 50. Death usually results within 15 years. Also called "Huntington's chorea".

Hydrocephaly: A defect marked by an unusual accumulation of spinal fluid in the ventricles of the brain. This fluid buildup usually retards brain development, often resulting in mental retardation and, in severe cases, early death. The condition can now be treated if diagnosed soon after birth.

Hypothalamus: A structure on the floor of one of the brain's fluid-filled cavities that is involved in the control of such homeostatic body functions as food and water intake, body temperature, heart rate, and blood pressure. It is part of a group of structures called the limbic system that influences sex drive, motivation, and emotional states. The hypothalamus exerts its influence through both the nervous and endocrine systems.

Immune: Protected against disease by innate or acquired (active or passive) immunity.

Immune system: A specialized group of body cells and cell products that respond to foreign organisms and substances in the body. The cell products are a.o. immunoglobulins (antibodies), produced by specialized white blood cells known as lymphocytes. Some lymphocytes and various other cells of the immune system directly attack foreign organisms or matter.

Immunity: The condition of being immune; an organism's capacity to resist disease. Immunity may be either innate or acquired. Innate immunity is natural or inherited. Acquired immunity may be active (resulting from either previous exposure to the disease-causing agent or vaccination) or passive (resulting from the transfer of preformed antibodies in immune serum or from mother to fetus).

Immunoassay: The use of antibodies to identify and quantify substances. The binding of antibodies to antigen, the substance being measured, is often accompanied by tracers such as radioisotopes.

Impairment: A physiological, anatomical, or mental loss or "abnormality" caused by accident, disease, or congenital condition. An impairment may be the underlying cause of a disability. Compare to **disability** and **handicap**.

Incidence: The frequency of new occurrences of a specific disease within a defined time interval. Incidence rate is the number of new cases of specified disease divided by the number of people in a population over a specified period of time, usually 1 year. Compare **prevalence**.

Inpatient care: Care that includes an overnight stay in a medical facility.

International Classification of Diseases, Ninth Revision, Clinical Modification (ICD-9-CM) Coding: A two-part system of coding patient medical information used in abstracting systems and for classifying patients into DRGs for Medicare. The first part is a comprehensive list of diseases with corresponding codes compatible with the World Health Organization's list of disease codes. The second part contains procedure codes, independent of the disease codes.

In vitro: Literally, "in glass", pertaining to a biological process or reaction taking place in an artificial environment, usually a laboratory. Sometimes used to include the growth of cells from multicellular organisms under cell culture conditions.

In vivo: Literally, "in the living", pertaining to a biological process or reaction taking place in a living cell or organism.

Lesion: Any abnormal discontinuity of tissue or loss of function. A wound, injury, or one of the individual points or patches of a multifocal disease.

Lipid metabolism: The process by which lipid (fatty) molecules are broken down or synthesized in the body.

Liposome: A structure with a lipid membrane like that of a cell which can be filled with specific substances and then used as a delivery vehicle transporting those substances to the interior of a target cell by fusion with the cell's own membrane. It is one of several potential delivery vehicles for use in gene therapy.

Manic depression: An illness whose symptoms include abnormal mood swings cycling from deep depression to uncontrollable feelings of elation (mania). It has unidentified genetic and biochemical components and is sometimes treatable with simple lithium salt.

Medical technology: The drugs, devices, and medical and surgical procedures used in medical care, and the organizational and support systems within which such care is provided.

Micro-organism: A minute, microscopic or submicroscopic living organism. Examples are bacteria, mycoplasma, viruses, and protozoa.

Molecular biology: The study of biology at the level of individual molecules, such as proteins and DNA.

Morbidity: 1. The condition of being diseased.
2. The ratio of sick to healthy persons in a community

Morphology: The study of the configuration or structure of organisms.

Mortality rate: The death rate, often made explicit for a particular characteristic, e.g., age, sex, or specific cause of death. A mortality rate contains three essential elements: 1) the number of people in a population group exposed to the risk of death; 2) a time factor; 3) the number of deaths occurring in the exposed population during a certain time period.

Multiple sclerosis: A progressive, crippling disease of unknown cause that destroys the myelin sheath that insulates nerve cell axons. This results in slowed nerve conduction. Symptoms commonly include muscle weakness, lack of coordination, as well as speech and visual disturbances.

Necrosis: Death of tissue.

Nerve block: Regional anaesthesia secured by making infections in close proximity to the nerve whose conductivity is to be cut off.

Neuroleptic: A term used to describe any drug (e.g., certain tranquilizers) useful in the treatment of mental disorders, especially psychoses.

Neuromodulator: Any substance, including hormones and neurotransmitters, that can regulate the strength of signaling between a neuron and another cell without acting directly on the receiving cell, either by regulating the amount of hormone present in the synapse or its receptor-binding capabilities.

Neuron: A nerve cell, the "active unit" of the nervous system and responsible for receiving and transmitting neural signals.

Neuropeptide: A general term for any peptide found in the central nervous system that affects the behavior of nerve cells, whether by acting as a neurotransmitter, hormone, or neuromodulator.

Neurosis: A variety of minor psychological disorders common in any population. Examples include obsessive-compulsive neurosis and phobias.

Neurotic: Referring to neurosis.

Neurotransmitter: A substance able to transfer a neural impulse across a synapse from one neuron to another, or from a neuron to an effector organ (e.g., a muscle or gland). An example is acetylcholine in the neuromuscular junction.

Noninvasive technique: A diagnostic method that does not involve the penetration (by surgery or hypodermic needle) of the skin.

Nuclear magnetic resonance: A phenomenon in which atoms can be induced, by use of a magnetic field, to emit energy. For diagnostic purposes this emitted energy can be "translated" into images of areas inside the living body.

Occlusion: In the context of the vascular system, the blocking off or obstruction of blood flow through a vessel.

Opiate: Any substance deriving from the opium poppy. Opiate drugs (e.g., morphine, heroin) bind to specific receptors on nerve cells scattered throughout the brain to reduce pain and produce euphoria. Repeated use of these agents is associated with biological tolerance and addiction. Naturally produced molecules (e.g., endorphin, encephalin) bind to the same nerve cell receptors and are called "endogenous" opiates or opioid drugs.

Outpatient care: Care provided in a hospital which does not include an overnight stay.

Palliative treatment: Treatment designed to provide relief from a disease or condition (e.g., to provide comfort or reduce pain), but not to cure the disease or condition.

Parkinson's disease: A disease affecting movement also leading to dementia, speech defects, and other neurological symptoms. The movement disorder is apparently due, in part, to degeneration of a group of cells in the substantia nigra in the brainstem. The reason for loss of these cells is not known.

Pathogen: A specific causative agent (e.g., a virus or bacterium) of a disease.

Pathogenesis: The mode of origin and development of a disease process.

Pathogenicity: The condition of causing disease.

Pathology: The scientific study of the cause of disease and of the associated structural and functional changes that are the result of disease.

Peptide: Compounds consisting of two or more amino acids linked together by a chemical process that produces one molecule of water for each joining of one amino acid to another. Peptides are the building blocks of proteins. Several peptides have recently been found to act as neurotransmitters.

Peripheral: Situated away from a center or central structure.

Phobia: Any persistent abnormal dread or fear.

Phosphorus NMR spectroscopy: A technique in which the individual components of the nuclear magnetic resonance (NMR) signals from phosphorous-containing compounds are analyzed according to frequency.

Pituitary gland: also called hypophysis. A gland located at th base of the brain, attached by a stalk to the hypothalamus, from which it receives an important neural outflow. It secretes several hormones of vital importance for growth, maturation, and reproduction of the individual.

Placebo: A drug or procedure with no intrinsic therapeutic value. In a randomized clinical trial, a placebo is given to patients in control groups as a means to blind investigators and patients alike as to whether an individual is receiving the experimental or the control treatment. This in order to avoid a biased interpretation of the resulting experimental data.

Placebo effect: An improvement in a condition that occurs in response to a placebo or treatment, but cannot be considered a result of the specific treatment used.

Polypeptide: A sequence of amino acids (at least three) joined in a chain.

Positron-emission tomography (PET): A noninvasive scanning technique measuring the uptake of radioactively labeled substances that emit subatomic particles (positrons). PET scans provide a dynamic picture of the brain's metabolic activity, as opposed to computed tomography (CT) scans, which yield a static anatomical view of parts of the brain.

Prevalence: In epidemiology, the number of cases of a specific disease, infected persons, or persons with disabilities or some other condition, present at a particular time and in relation to the size of the population. Also called "prevalence rate". Compare **incidence**.

Prevention: See **disease prevention.**

Procedure (medical or surgical): A medical technology involving any combination of drugs, devices, and provider skills and abilities. Appendectomy, for example, may involve at least drugs (for anesthesia), monitoring devices, surgical devices, and the skilled actions of physicians, nurses, and support staffs.

Prosthesis: An artificial substitute for a missing body part such as an arm or a leg.

Protein: A polypeptide consisting of amino acids. In their biologically active states, they function as catalysts in metabolism and as structural elements of cells and tissues.

Psychopharmaceutical: A term used to describe drugs that affect mental function.

Psychosis: A general term for any major mental illness characterized by personality disorders, loss of contact with reality, and sometimes delusions or hallucinations.

Psychotropic: Exerting an effect on mental activity; the term is usually applied to drugs that affect the mental state.

Random allocation: In a randomized clinical trial, allocation of individuals to treatment groups in such a way that each individual has an equal probability of being assigned to any group.

Randomized clinical trial (RCT): An experiment, designed to test the safety and efficacy of a medical technology, in which people are randomly allocated to experimental or control groups, and outcomes are compared.

Receptor: A protein embedded in the cell membrane to which a neurotransmitter or other specific molecule can bind to excite or inhibit activity of the cell. An example is the acetylcholine receptor in muscle cells.

Recombinant DNA (rDNA) technology: Techniques involving the incorporation of DNA fragments, generated with the use of restriction enzymes, into a suitable host organism's DNA (a vector). The host is then grown in culture to produce clones with multiple copies of the incorporated DNA fragment. The clones containing this particular DNA fragment can then be selected and harvested.

Regeneration: Repair or regrowth of a cell, tissue, or structure.

Releasing factors: Factors (chemically uncharacterized hormones) secreted by the hypothalamus that trigger the pituitary gland to release certain hormones (e.g., growth hormone releasing factor).

Risk: 1) A measure of the probability of an adverse or untoward outcome and the severity of the resultant harm to health of individuals in a defined population and associated with the use of a medical technology applied for a given medical problem under specified conditions of use. 2) The predicted or observed effects of exposure to toxic substances or harmful physical agents in the workplace, general environment, consumer products, etc.

Safety: A judgment of the acceptability of risk in a specified situation. See also **Risk**.

Schizophrenia: Any of a group of severe psychiatric disorders characterized by a.o. misinterpretation and retreat from reality, withdrawal, hallucination, and bizarre or regressive behavior.. Some forms of schizophrenia seem to involve genetic and biochemical abnormalities--possibly involving an excess of dopamine or imbalances of other neurotransmitters in certain brain regions. The term "schizophrenia" should not be confused with "multiple personality".

Sensitivity: The true positive ratio. In referring to a diagnostic test, it is the extent to which abnormals are correctly classified.

Somatic: A term used to refer to body tissues apart from reproductive (germinal) tissues.

Specificity: The true negative ratio. In referring to a diagnostic test, it is the extent to which normals are correctly classified. Compare **sensitivity**.

Stroke: Loss of function due to inadequate circulation of blood in the brain caused by sudden lesions in the blood vessels of the brain. This can be caused by heart failure, blockage of arteries or veins, or bleeding into the brain. This condition is often followed by permanent neurological damage.

Substantia nigra: A darkly pigmented structure in the brain containing a group of neurons that use dopamine as their transmitter in their connection with the basal ganglia (a structure involved in the coordination and initiation of movement). A deficit of dopamine in these connections is characteristic of Parkinson's disease and produces its motor symptoms. See **Parkinson's disease**.

Synapse: An area across which signals are transmitted from the axon ending of a nerve cell to the membrane of an adjacent neuron or effector cell (e.g. muscle or gland cell). Synapses may be "chemical", using a neurotransmitter to transmit the signal across a small gap between the membranes, or "electrical", in which the neuron's cytoplasm is actually joined with that of the adjacent cell, forming a bridge or "gap junction".

Technology: The application of organized knowledge to practical ends.

Technology assessment: In general, a comprehensive form of policy research that examines the technical, economic, and social consequences of technological applications. It is especially concerned with unintended, indirect, or delayed social impacts. In health policy, however, the term more often is used to mean any form of policy analysis concerned with medical technology, especially the evaluation of efficacy and safety. The comprehensive form of technology assessment is then termed "comprehensive technology assessment".

Technology diffusion: The diffusion or spread of a medical technology into the health care system. It is generally thought to be in two phases: the initial phase in which decisions are made to adopt or reject the technology, and a subsequent phase in which decisions are made to use the technology.

Therapeutic technology: A technology that cures or relieves the symptoms of a disease or other medical condition.

Thrombosis: The formation, development, or presence of a solid mass in a blood vessel or in the heart. It is composed of fibrin, platelets, and, in most instances, erythrocytes.

Tomographic scan: The image of one selected layer or plane of the body.

Transient ischemic attack: A deficiency of blood in a part of the body (typically the brain) due to functional constriction or actual obstruction of a blood vessel.

Transplantation: With respect to human organs, the transplanting of a healthy organ (e.g., kidney, cornea, liver, and so on) from a donor, living or recently deceased, into a patient with absent or inadequate functioning of the equivalent organ.

Validity: A measure of the extent to which an observed situation reflects the "true" situation. Internal validity is a measure of the extent to which study results reflect the true relationship of a technology to the outcome of interest in the study subjects. External validity is a measure of the extent to which study results can be generalized to the population which in the study is represented by individuals.

Virology: The study of viruses.

Virulence: The degree and severity with which a pathogen is able to infect a population and cause disease.

Virus: Any of a large group of submicroscopic agents infecting plants, animals, and bacteria and characterized by a total dependence on living cells for reproduction and by a lack of independent metabolism. A fully formed virus consists of nucleic acid (DNA or RNA) surrounded by a protein or protein and lipid coat.

APPENDIX E GLOSSARY OF ACRONYMS

ACTH	Adrenocorticotrophic hormone
ALS	Amyotrophic lateral sclerosis
AMP	Adenosine mono phosphate
BBB	Blood brain barrier
CA^{++}	Calcium ions
CAM	Cell adhesive molecule
CNS	Central nervous system
CT	Computed tomography
cDNA	Complementary deoxyribonucleic acid
DA	Dopamine
DNA	Deoxyribonucleic acid
DOPA	Dihydroxyphenylalanine
ECT	Electro convulsive treatment
EEG	Electroencephalography
GABA	Gamma aminobutyric acid
GAP	Growth-associated protein
GM1	Monosialoganglioside
HLA	Human leukocyte antigen
LTP	Long term potentiation
MEG	Magnetoencephalography
MPTP	1-Methyl-4-phenyl-1,2,5,6-tetrahydropyridine
MRI	Magnetic resonance imaging
mRNA	Messenger ribonucleic acid
MRS	Magnetic resonance spectroscopy
MS	Multiple sclerosis
MSH	Melanotropin
N-CAM	Neural cell adhesive molecule
NGF	Nerve growth factor
NMDA	N-methyl-D-aspartate (a type of receptor)
NMR	Nuclear magnetic resonance
NPF	Neurite-promoting factor
NTF	Neurotrophic factor
PET	Positron emission tomography
PNS	Peripheral nervous system
POMC	Pro-opiomelanocortin
PVN	Paraventricular nucleus
RNA	Ribonucleic acid
SDAT	Senile dementia of the Alzheimer's type
SON	Supraoptic nucleus
STG	Stuurgroep Toekomstscenario's Gezondheidszorg (The Steering Committee on Future Health Scenarios)
VIP	Vasoactive intestinal peptide

APPENDIX F REFERENCES

1. Anderson B. Is alpha-MSH deficiency the cause of Alzheimer's disease? Medical Hypotheses 1986; 19: 379-385.

2. Anderson DW, Miller JD, Kalsbeek WD. Findings from a major U.S. survey of persons hospitalized with head injuries. Public Health Reports 1983; 98: 475-478.

3. Appel SH, Ojika K, Tomozawa Y, Bostwick R. Trophic factors in brain aging and disease. In: Traber J, Gispen WH (eds.). Senile dementia of the alzheimer's type, early diagnosis, neuropathology and animal models. Berlin Heidelberg, West-Germany: Springer-Verlag, 1985: 218-230.

4. Arima M, Suzuki Y, Yabuuchi H. The developing brain and its disorders. Tokyo: University of Tokyo Press, 1984.

5. Barnes DM. Nervous and immune system disorders linked in a variety of diseases. Science 1986; 232: 160-161.

6. Barnes DM. Brain architecture: beyond genes. Science 1986; 233: 155-156.

7. Barranger JA, Brady RO (eds.). Molecular basis of lysosomal storage disorders. Orlando, United States: Academic Press, inc., 1984.

8. Beattie M, Stokes B, Bresnahan J, Somerson S. Anatomical, behavioral and physiological studies of controlled spinal cord injury. In: Sabel B, Stein DG (eds.). Pharmacological approaches to the treatment of brain and spinal cord injury. Baton Rouge, Louisiana: Louisiana State University Press, 1987 (in press).

9. de Beaufort I. Ethiek en medische experimenten met mensen; proefschrift. Rijksuniversiteit Groningen, 1985.

10. Bercsy I (ed). Pituitary function and immunuty. CRC press, Boca Raton, Florida, 1986.

11. Bjorklund A, Gage, FH. Neuronal replacement after traumatic or age-dependent brain damage: a review of experimental work in rodents and its clinical implications. International Journal of Technology Assessment in Health Care 1985; 1: 93 -107.

12. Bjorklund A, Stefenevi U. Intracerebral neural implants: neuronal replacement and reconstruction of damaged circuitries. Annual Review on Neurosciences 1984; 7: 279-308.

13. Blalock JE, Harbous-Mc.Menamyn D, Smith EM. Peptide hormones shared by the neuro-endocrine and immunologic systems. Journal of Immunology 1985; 135: 858-861 (supplement).

14. Bloom FE. Neurotransmitters and CNS disease: the future. The Lancet 1982; 2: 1381-1385.

15. Bloom FE, Lazerson A, Hofstadter L. Brain, mind and behavior. New York: W.H. Freeman and Company, 1985.

16. Bocchetta A, Corsini GU. Parkinson's disease and pesticides. The Lancet 1986; 2: 1163.

17. Bower B. Tracking the roots of Parkinson's disease. Science News 1985; 128: 212.

18. Te Braake ThAM. In vitro fertilisatie en wetenschappelijk onderzoek op embryo's. Tijdschrift voor Gezondheidsrecht 1985; 9: 247-248.

19. Brody JA, White LR. Risk factors for senile dementia. In: Rotshild H (ed.). Risk factors for senility. Oxford, United Kingdom: Oxford University Press, 1984.

20. Brown CE, Battocletti IH, Johnson LF. Nuclear magnetic resonance (NMR) in clinical pathology: current trends. Clinical Chemistry 1984; 30: 606-618.

21. Brown MC, Holland RL, Hopkins WG. Motor nerve sprouting. In: Cowan WM, Hall ZW, Kandel ER. Annual Revieuw of Neuroscience 1981; 4: 17-42.

22. Brown MR, Fisher LA. Brain peptides as intercellular messengers, implications for medicine. JAMA 1984; 251: 1310-1315.

23. Budinger TF, Lauterbur PC. Nuclear magnetic resonance technology for medical studies. Science 1984; 226: 288-298.

24. Calne DB, McGeer E, Eisen A, Spencer P. Alzheimer's disease, Parkinson's disease, and motoneurone disease: abiotropic interaction between ageing and environment? The Lancet 1986; 2: 1067-1070.

25. Calne DB, Langston JW. Aethiology of Parkinson's disease. The Lancet 1983; 2: 1457-1459.

26. Canadian Journal of Neurological Sciences 1984, 11.1, Supplement: 89-237.

27. Charatan FB. Mental stimulation and deprivation as risk factors in Senility. In: Rotshild H (ed.). Risk factors for senility. Oxford, United Kingdom: Oxford University Press, 1984.

28. Collingridge GL, Kehl SJ, McLennan H. Excitatory aminoacids in synaptic transmission in the collateral-commissural pathway of the lateral hippocampus. Journal of Physiology 1983; 334: 33-46.

29. Committee on Science, Engineering and Public Policy of the National Academy of Sciences, National Academy of Engineering and Institute of Medicine. Outlook for science and technology: the next five years, volume III. Washington D.C.: National Academy Press, 1982.

30. Condon B, Wyper D, Grant R, Patterson J, Hadley D, Teasdale G, Rowan J. Use of magnetic resonance imaging to measure intracranial cerebrospinal fluid volume. The Lancet 1986; 2: 1355-1357.

31. Cools AR, Jaspers R, Schwarz M, Sontag KH, Vrijmoed-de Vries M, Van den Bercken J. Basal ganglia and switching motor programs. In: J.S. McKenzie, R.E. Kemm, and L.N. Wilcock (Eds.). The basal ganglia. New York: Plenum Publishing Corporation, 1984 pp. 513-544.

32. Cotman CW, Nieto-Sampedro M. Progress in facilitating the recovery of function after central nervous system trauma. Annals New York Academy of Sciences 1985; 181: 83-104.

33. Crawford DIO, Harris R. Ethics of predictive testing for Huntington's Chorea: the need for more information. British Medical Journal 1986; 293: 249-251.

34. Cullen JM, Spadaro JA. Axonal regenerarion in the spinal cord: a role for applied electricity. Journal of Bioelectricity 1983; 2: 57-75.

35. Dakof GA, Mendelsohn GA. Parkinson's disease: the psychological aspects of a chronic illness. Psychological Bulletin 1986; 99: 375-387.

36. Davis J. Endorphins: new waves in brain chemistry. New York, United States: The Dial Press, 1984.

37. Davis KL, Mohs RC. Cholinergic drugs in Alzheimer's disease. The New England Journal of Medicine 1986; 315: 1286-1287.

38. Declaration of Helsinki. World Medical Association, 1975.

39. Edwards PM, Gispen WH. Melanocortin peptides and neural plasticity, In; Traber J, Gispen WH, (eds.). Senile dementia of the Alzheimer's type, early diagnosis, neuropathology and animal models. Berlin Heidelberg, Germany: Springer-Verlag, 1985.

40. Edwards PM, Kuiters RRF, Boer GJ, Gispen WH. Recovery from peripheral nerve transection is accelerated by local application of a-MSH by means of microporous accurel(r) polypropylene tubes. Journal of the Neurological Sciences 1986; 74: 171-176.

41. Elliot GR, Eisdorfer C, eds. Stress and human health: analysis and implications of research. New York: Springer Publishing Company, 1982.

42. Felten DL, Felten SY, Carlson SL, Olschowka JA, Livnat S. Noradrenergic and peptidergic innervation of lymphoid tissue. Journal of Immunology 1985; 135: 755-765 (supplement).

43. Finch C. Comments on reviews by Gash et.al. Applications of recombinant DNA techniques. Neurobiology of Ageing 1985; 6: 156-157.

44. Fine A. Peptides and Alzheimer's disease. Nature 1986; 319: 537-538.

45. Fine A. Transplantation in the central nervous system. Scientific American 1986; 255: 42-50.

46. Fine PR. Kuhlemeier KV, De Vivo MJ, Stover SL. Spinal cord injury: an epidemilogic perspective. Paraplegia 1979-1980; 17: 237-250.

47. Fishman PS. Neuronal transplantation: scientific gains and clinical perspectives. Neurology 1986; 36: 389-392.

48. Fishman PS, Gass JS, Swoveland PT, Lavi E, Highkin MK, Weiss SR. Infection of the basal ganglia by a murine coronavirus. Science 1985; 229: 877-879.

49. Frederiks JAM. Dementie. Nederlands Tijdschrift voor de Geneeskunde 1985; 129: 2199-2205.

50. Freed WJ. Repairing neuronal circuits with brain grafts: where can brain grafts be used as a therapy? Neurobiology of Aging 1985; 6: 153-156.

51. Freed WJK, de Medinaceli L, Wyatt RJK. Promoting functional plasticity in the damaged nervous system. Science 1985; 227: 1544-1552.

52. Gage FH, Bjorklund A. Problems specifically related to grafting to the aged brain. Neurobiology of Ageing 1985; 6: 163-164.

53. Galjaard H. Onderzoek van foetaal weefsel: mag dat? Nederlands Tijdschrift voor de Geneeskunde 1984; 128: 2276-2277.

54. Garruto RM, Swyt C, Yanagihara R, Fiori CE, Gajdusek DC. Intraneuronal co-localization of silicon with calcium and aluminium in amyotrophic lateral sclerosis and parkinsonism with dementia of guam. The New England Journal of Medicine 1986; 315: 711.

55. Gash DM, Collier TJ, Sladek JR. Neural transplantation: a review of recent developments and potential applications to the aged brain. Neurobiology of Aging 1985; 6: 131-150.

56. Geisler WO, Jousse AT, Wynne-Jones M, Breithaupt D. Survival in traumatic spinal cord injury. Paraplegia 1983; 21: 364 -373.

57. Gezondheidsraad. Advies inzake het gebruik van foetussen, foetaal weefsel of andere stoffelijke resten na abortus, voor wetenschappelijke doeleinden. The Hague, The Netherlands, 1984.

58. Gezondheidsraad. Advies inzake magnetische resonantie spectroscopie. The Hague, The Netherlands, 1986.

59. Gezondheidsraad. Advies inzake teratogeniteit van chemische stoffen. The Hague, The Netherlands, 1985.

60. Gillin JC, Borbely AA. Sleep: a neurobiological window on affective disorders. Trends in Neurosciences 1985; 8: 537.

61. Gjone R, Nordlie L. Incidence of traumatic paraplegia and tetraplegia in Norway: a statistical survey of the years 1974 and 1975. Paraplegia 1978-1979; 16: 88-89.

62. Goldstein GW, Betz AL. The blood brain barrier. Scientific American 1986; 255: 70-80.

63. Green J. Detecting the hypersusceptible worker: genetics and politics in industrial medicine. International Journal of Health Services 1983; 13: 247-264.

64. Guth L, Barnett CP, Donati EJ, Smith MV, Lifson M, Roberts E. Enhancement of axonal growth into a spinal lesion by topical application of triethanolamine and cytosine arabinoside. Experimental Neurology 1985; 88: 44-55.

65. Hellegers AE. Fetal research. In: Reich WT (ed.). Encyclopedia of bioethics, New York: The Free Press, 1978: 489-493.

66. Hubel DH, Wiesel TN. The period of susceptibility to the physiological effects of unilateral eye closure in kittens. Journal of Physiology 1970; 206: 419-436.

67. Hyman MD. Sociopsychological obstacles to L-DOPA therapy that may limit effectiveness in parkinsonism. Journal of the American Geriatric Society 1972; 20: 200-208.

68. Jolles J. Vasopressin and cognitive performance in man. In: Psychiatry: the state of the art, vol V: child and addolescent psychiatry. New York: Plenum Publishing Corporation, 1985: 327-332.

69. Jolles J. Early diagnosis of dementia. Possible contributions of neuropsychology. In: Traber J and Gispen WH (eds.). Senile dementia of the Alzheimer type, early diagnosis, neuropathology and animal models. Berlin: Springer Verlag, 1985: 84-100.

70. Jolles J. Cognitive, emotional and behavioral dysfunctions in aging and dementia. Progression in Brain Research 1986; 70: 15-39.

71. Kandel B, Schwarz JH. Principles of Neuro Sciences 2nd. ed. Amsterdam: Elzevier Publishing Co., 1985.

72. Katzman R. The prevalence and malignancy of Alzheimer's disease- a major killer. Archives of Neurology 1976; 33: 217-218.

73. Kay DWK, Bergmann K. Epidemiology of mental disorders among the aged in the community. In: Birren JE. Handbook of Mental Health and Aging 1980; 34-56.

74. Karpiak S, Vilim F, Mahadik SP. Ganglioside effects on neuronal plasticity during development. Neurotoxicology 1986; 1: 350.

75. Kety SS. Disorders of the human brain. Scientific American 1979; 241: 172-180.

76. Kolata G. Researchers hunt for Alzheimer's disease gene. Science 1986; 232: 448-450.

77. Kolb B, Whishaw IQ. Fundamentals of human neuropsychology. San Francisco: WH Freeman and Co, 1985.

78. Kraus JF, Black MA, Hessol N, Ley P, Rokaw W, Sullivan C, Bowers S, Knowlton S, Marshall L. The incidence of acute brain injury and serious impairment in a defined population. American Journal of Epidemiology 1984; 119: 186-201.

79. Langston JW, Ballard P, Tetrud JW, Irwin I. Chronic Parkinsonism in humans due to a product of meperidine-analog synthesis. Science 1983; 219: 979-980.

80. Lebacqz K, Levine RJ. Informed consent in human research: ethical and legal aspects. In: Reich WT (ed.). Encyclopedia of Bioethics, New York: The Free Press, 1978: 754-762.

81. Leenen HJJ. Gezondheidszorg en recht: een gezondheidsrechtelijke studie, Alphen aan de Rijn: Samson, 1981.

82. Lezak MD. Neuropsychological assessment, 2nd edn. New York: Oxford University Press, 1983.

83. Little JW, Halar E. Temporal course of motor recovery after brown-sequard spinal cord injuries. Paraplegia 1985; 23 :39 -46.

84. Lopes da Silva FH. Hippocampal kidling: physiological evidence for progressive disinhibition. In: Wolf P and Janz CE (eds.). Advances in Epileptology. New York: Raven Press 1986; 16: chap. 12.

85. Lorenz K. The comparative method of studying innate behaviour patterns. Symp. Soc. exp. Biol. 1950; 4: 229-269.

86. Martin JB, Gusella JF. Huntington's disease, pathogenesis and management. The New England Journal of Medicine 1986; 315: 1267-1276.

87. Marx JL. Nerve growth factor acts in brain. Science 1986; 232: 1341-1342.

88. Medical World News. Regenerating damaged peripheral nerves. 1985; 26: 4.

89. Meinardi. Inaugural lecture University of Nijmegen, 1985.

90. Minaire P, Castenier M, Girard R, Berard E, Deidier C, Bourret J. Epidemiology of spinal cord injury in the Rhone-Alpes region, France, 1970-1975. Paraplegia 1978-1979; 16: 76-87.

91. Minderhoud JM, Blandeau-Middendorp J, Boelens MEM, Brouwers OF, Wisman HP, Van Kerkvoorde RJ, Snijder BR, Bollen MAAJ, Bijleveld TJ, Masselink HG, Van Vlokhoven TAM. Epidemiologie van schedel-hersenletsel in de regio Groningen: analyse van verkeersongevallen in 1971-1972, 1974-1975, en 1977-1978. Tijdschrift voor Sociale Geneeskunde 1980; 58: 622-630.

92. Mirmiran M, van Gool WA, van Haaren F, Polak CE. Environmental influences on brain and behavior in aging and senile dementia. Progress in Brain Research 1986; 70: 443-460.

93. Morris RGM, Hagan JJ, Rawlins JNP. Allocentric spatial learning by hippocampectomized rats: a further test of the "spatial mapping" and "working memory" theories of hippocampal function. Quarterly Journal of Experimental Psychology Section B Comparative And Physiological Psychology 1986; 38: 365-396.

94. Mulley GP. Differential diagnosis of dementia. British Medical Journal 1986; 292: 1416-1418.

95. National commission for the protection of human subjects of biomedical and behavioral research: report on research on the fetus to the secretary. Department of Health, Education, and Welfare, 1975.

96. National Institute of Mental Health. The neurosciences of mental health: a report on neuroscience research. DHHS publication no. (adm) 85-1363. Rockville, Maryland, 1984.

97. Nelson EL, Melton J, Annegers JF, Laws ER, Offord KP. Incidence of skull fractures in Olmsted county, Minnesota. Neurosurgery 1984; 15: 318-323.

98. Nottebohm F. A brain for all seasons: cyclical anatomical changes

in song control nuclei of the canary brain. Science 1981; 214: 1368-1370.

99. Office of Technology Assessment. Impacts of neuroscience. Washington, DC: US Government Printing Office, 1985.

100. Phelps ME, Mazziotta JC. Positron emission tomography: human brain function and biochemistry. Science 1985; 228: 799-809.

101. President's Commission for the study of Ethical Problems in Medicine and Biomedical and Behavioral research. Summing up; the ethical and legal problems in medicine and biomedical and behavioural research, New York, 1983.

102. Pritchard JW, Schulman RG. NMR-spectroscopy of brain metabolism in vivo. Annual Revieuws of Neuroscience 1986; 9: 61-81.

103. Raichle ME. Positron emission tomography. Annual Reviews of Neuroscience 1983; 6: 249-267.

104. Raymond CA. In pursuit of quarry, MS researchers draw on immunology, virology advances. Journal of the American Medical Association 1986; 256: 809-816.

105. Redmond DE, Roth RH, Elsworth JD, Sladek JR, Collier TJK, Deutch AY, Haber S. Fetal neuronal grafts in monkeys given methylphenyltetrahydropyridine. The Lancet 1986; 1: 1125-1127.

106. Reier PJ. Neural tissue grafts and repair of the injured spinal cord. Neuropathology and Applied Neurobiology 1985; 11: 81-104.

107. Roscam Abbing. Genetische experimenten met mensen. Medisch Contact 1986; 17: 533-535.

108. Rutishauer U. Molecular and biological properties of a neural cell adhesion molecule. Symposium on Quantitative Biology 1983; 48: 501-514.

109. Sabel BA. Treating brain injury with gangliosides. Integrative Psychiatry 1985; 3: 199-210.

110. Sabel BA, Stein DG. Pharmacological treatment of central nervous system injury. Nature 1986; 323: 493.

111. Sanes JR, Covault J. Axon guidance during reinnervation of skeletal muscle. Trends in Neurosciences 1985; 8: 103-105.

112. Singer E. Sociopsychological factors influencing response to levodopa therapy for Parkinson's disease. Archives of Physical Medicine and Rehabilitation 1976; 57: 328-334.

113. Singh R. Histocompatibility matching and preserved nerve allografts in dogs (dissertation). Rotterdam, 1983.

114. Slack JR, Hopkins WG, Pockett S. Evidence for a motor nerve growth factor. Muscle Nerve 1983; 6: 243-252.

115. Sperry RW. Science and moral priority: merging mind, brain and human values. New York: Columbia University Press, 1983.

116. Stahl SM, Leenders KL, Bowery NG. Imaging neurotransmitters and their receptors in living human brain by positron emission tomography. Trends in Neurosciences 1986; 9: 241-145.

117. Stein DG. Fetal brain tissue transplant techniques: a cautionary note. Neurobiology of Ageing 1985; 6: 157-160.

118. Stern GM, Lander CM, Lees AJ. Akinetic freezing and trick movements in Parkinson's disease. Journal of Neural Transmission 1980; 16: 137-141.

119. Stuurgroep Toekomstscenarios Gezondheidszorg (STG). Accidents and traumatology. The Hague, 1986 draft.

120. Stuurgroep Toekomstscenarios Gezondheidszorg (STG). Ouder worden in de toekomst. Scenarios over gezondheid en vergrijzing 1984-2000. The Hague, 1984.

121. Swaab DF, Fliers E. Clinical strategies in the treatment of Alzheimer's disease. Netherlands Institute for Brain Research, 1985.

122. Task Force on Basic Science, Report to the National Advisory Neurological and Communicative Disorders and Stroke Council, NIH Publication no. 79-1920, Washington D.C., 1979.

123. Ter-Pogossian MM, Raichle ME, Sotel BE. Positron Emission Tomography. Scientific American 1980; 243: 140-156.

124. Toffano G, Leon A. Central nervous system repair and nerve cell cultures. Pharmacological Research Communications 1986; 18: 187-201.

125. Toffano G, Savoini G, Aldinio C, Valenti G, Dal Taso R, Leon A, Calza L, Zini J, Agnati LF, Fuxe K. Effects of gangliosides on the functional recovery of damaged brain. Advances in Experimental Medical Biology 1984; 174: 475-488.

126. Traber J, Gispen W.H. (eds.). Senile dementia of the Alzheimer's type, early diagnosis, neuropathology and animal models. Berlin Heidelberg: Springer-Verlag, 1985.

127. Turk R, Obreza P. Functional electrical stimulation as an orthotic means for the rehabilitation of paraplegic patients. Paraplegia 1985; 23: 344-348.

128. Varon S. Factors promoting the growth of the nervous system. Neurosciences 1985; 3: 62.

129. De Wied D. The neuropeptide concept. Maturitas 1984; 6: 217-223.

130. Willard M, Skene P. Molecular extents in axonal regeneration. In: Nicholls JG (ed.). Repair and regeneration of the nervous system. Heidelberg: Springer-Verlag, 1982: 71-89.

APPENDIX G ACKNOWLEDGEMENTS

Contractors and Consultants

Prof. dr. W.H. Gispen and prof. dr. F.H. Lopes da Silva drafted Chapter II, the Regeneration, Repair and Reorganization of Nervous Tissue, of this report. Furthermore, they reviewed all written materials. Prof. dr. W.H. Gispen also assisted in the set-up of the study and supported the staff in many valuable ways.

Chapter I of this report, Some Promising Directions of Research and Technology Development in Neurosciences, is based upon written contributions of the following authors:

Prof. dr. R.E.P.A. Ballieux
Academisch Ziekenhuis Utrecht

Prof. dr. B. Bohus
Rijksuniversiteit Groningen

Prof. dr. A.R. Cools
Katholieke Universiteit Nijmegen

Prof. dr. R.H. van den Hoofdakker
Academisch Ziekenhuis Groningen

Dr. F.G.I. Jennekens
Academisch Ziekenhuis Utrecht

Prof. dr. J. Jolles
Rijksuniversiteit Limburg

Prof. dr. T.D. Kernell
Academisch Medisch Centrum Amsterdam

Prof. dr. J. Korf
Academisch Ziekenhuis Groningen

Prof. dr. F.H. Lopes da Silva
Universiteit van Amsterdam

Dr. J.M. van Ree
Rudolph Magnus Instituut voor Farmacologie
Rijksuniversiteit Utrecht

Prof. dr. P.E. Voorhoeve
Academisch Medisch Centrum Amsterdam

Prof. dr. D. de Wied
Rudolph Magnus Instituut voor Farmacologie
Rijksuniversiteit Utrecht

Working Group on Medical Implications of Neurosciences Research (June 1986)

Prof. dr. A.R. Cools
Katholieke Universiteit Nijmegen

Prof. dr. W.H. Gispen
Rijksuniversiteit Utrecht

Dr. F.G.I. Jennekens
Academisch Ziekenhuis Utrecht

Dr. H.G.M. Rigter
Gezondheidsraad
s-Gravenhage

Prof. dr. F.H. Lopes da Silva
Universiteit van Amsterdam

Prof. dr. D.F. Swaab
Instituut voor Hersenonderzoek
Amsterdam

Working Group on Neurosciences (September 1985)

Prof. dr. R. Giel
Academisch Ziekenhuis Groningen

Prof. dr. W.H. Gispen
Rijksuniversiteit Utrecht

Prof. dr. H.J. van der Helm
Academisch Medisch Centrum Amsterdam

Dr. F.G.I. Jennekens
Academisch Ziekenhuis Utrecht

Prof. dr. T.D. Kernell
Academisch Medisch Centrum Amsterdam

Prof. dr. J. Korf
Academisch Ziekenhuis Groningen

Prof. dr. S.W.J. Lamberts
Academisch Ziekenhuis Rotterdam

Dr. J.M. van Ree
Rudolph Magnus Instituut voor Farmacologie
Rijksuniversiteit Utrecht

Dr. J.J. de Ridder
Organon International B.V.
Oss

Dr. D.J.B. Ringoir
Ministerie van Welzijn, Volksgezondheid en Cultuur
Geneeskundige Hoofdinspectie voor de Geestelijke Volksgezondheid

Mrs. prof. mr. H.D.C. Roscam Abbing
Rijksuniversiteit Limburg

Prof. dr. P.F. Voorhoeve
Academisch Medisch Centrum Amsterdam

www.ingramcontent.com/pod-product-compliance
Ingram Content Group UK Ltd.
Pitfield, Milton Keynes, MK11 3LW, UK
UKHW020148290926
15471UKWH00004B/753
* 9 7 8 0 8 9 8 3 8 4 1 9 2 *